Global Rituals

A Guide to Beauty, Self-Care, and Fragrance Traditions Around the World

NADIA KESSYN

SOFT CORNER
PUBLISHING

For permission requests, please contact:
Soft Corner Publishing™
Softcornerpublishing.com
info@softcornerpublishing.com

The author of this book does not dispense medical advice or prescribe the use of any technique as a form of treatment for physical, emotional, or medical problems without the advice of a physician or other qualified health-care professional. The information presented is offered for general informational purposes only and is not intended to replace professional medical advice, diagnosis, or treatment. Always seek the guidance of a qualified health professional with any questions you may have regarding a medical condition, skincare concern, allergic reaction, or the use of any product. Any application of the information in this book is undertaken at the reader's own discretion and sole risk. The author and publisher assume no responsibility for any outcome arising from the use of information contained herein.

ISBN: 979-8-9941765-1-1
Interior and cover design by
Soft Corner Publishing
Printed in the United States of America.

For my son,
who reminds me every day that care, curiosity,
and kindness are rituals too.
This is for you, and for the world you're
growing into.

4 | Global Rituals

Table of Contents

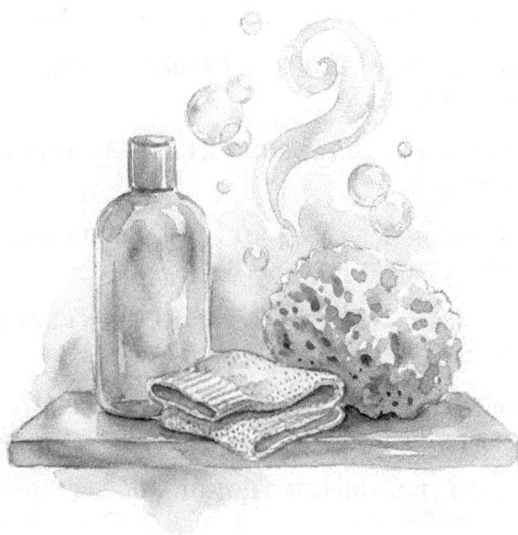

INTRODUCTION

Beauty as Ritual, Ritual as Belonging

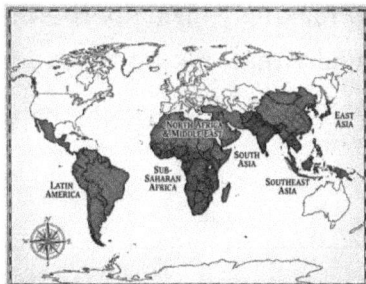

Picture this: steam rising in a bathhouse as someone pours water over their hair. Somewhere else, a woman mixes turmeric and sandalwood, humming a tune from her grandmother. These are both routines and stories. Every beauty ritual is a way of passing something down, one person to the next. It's a simple act, but it connects you to your past and gives your day a little more meaning.

Everywhere you look, people have their own ways of washing up, getting ready, and smelling good. These habits can help you feel better. They can bring people together. Whether you're in a crowded city salon or a small village bathhouse, these routines are a way of saying, 'I belong here.'

Sometimes, these routines even take you back. Maybe jasmine oil reminds you of bedtime as a kid. Rose water brings you back to a sunny celebration. These habits aren't just about looking good. They're about feeling calm, taking care of yourself, and making your daily routine feel like a small, personal ritual. It's a way to feel at home, wherever you are.

In the next chapters, we're heading into bathhouses in North Africa, kitchens in South Asia, and saunas in Northern Europe. You'll see how people in different places wash up, glow, and smell amazing, and how these old-school routines are popping up in bathrooms today. You'll find out what makes a Moroccan hammam so refreshing, how a South Asian ubtan can lift your mood, and why a Korean Italy (exfoliating) towel wakes you up fast. You'll even get a taste of the calm you find in a Japanese onsen.

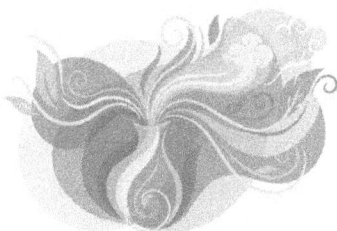

We'll also check out what's trending right now. TikTok hacks, global mashups, and the comeback of natural ingredients. A lot of what's new is pretty old. These viral routines usually have deep roots.

This book is your invitation to try out beauty traditions from around the world, with an open mind and a little respect. It's not rushed or complicated. You'll get stories, background, and real tips you can use at home. Want to mix up a simple ubtan mask? Set up a mini-hammam in your bathroom? Use an African exfoliating net? Layer oils and perfumes like a pro? You'll find all of that here.

It's just a way to bring a little bit of the world into your own routine.

You get a window into what matters to people everywhere. You start to see the care and creativity in every little habit. You might even look at your own routines in a new way. As a chance to take care of yourself and feel better, not just another thing to check off your list.

So get comfortable. Maybe grab something that smells nice. We're about to travel from continent to continent, from old traditions to new trends, and see how people everywhere use these routines to feel good inside and out. You'll see how a simple bath can change your mood, how a scent can hold a whole culture, and how washing up is not just getting clean.

Let's begin.

CHAPTER 1: SOUTH ASIA

Ancient Traditions in Modern Glow

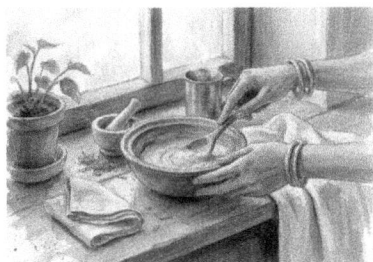

Imagine a courtyard in Jaipur. The sun casts a gentle warmth as a mom sits behind her daughter, rubbing coconut oil between her palms. The oil slips through her fingers, warm and smooth, before she works it into her daughter's hair. Next to them, a bowl filled with chickpea flour, turmeric, and rosewater sits ready. It's *ubtan* day, a tradition older than anyone can remember. The daughter closes her eyes and absorbs it all—the oil, her mom's nurturing touch, and the sun's gentle embrace on her back. This care is kept alive through familiar hands.

Traditional Rituals and Remedies

In South Asia, beauty doesn't start at the store. It starts in the kitchen, the garden, or while someone tells you a story and braids your hair. Ayurveda and other old wellness systems saw self-care as both medicine and devotion. Taking care of your body and your mind? Same thing. People just did it in a hundred different ways, from the mountains up north to the humid coasts down south.

Take the oil bath, for example. It goes by a lot of names, but everyone knows the feeling. Warm oil—sometimes with herbs or flowers—gets massaged into your skin and scalp. Sure, it's practical. Coconut, sesame, mustard, or almond oil all help your hair and skin handle tough weather. But honestly, the best part is how it makes you feel. A slow massage relaxes your muscles, calms your mind, and just makes everything feel a little easier.

In a lot of families, oiling your hair is a weekend thing. Elders sit you down, throw an old towel over your shoulders, and get to work. People tell stories, settle arguments, and someone always yells that tea is ready. Even now, people in busy cities still sneak in a scalp massage at the salon or oil their hair before bed. The bottles look different, but the habit hasn't changed.

After oiling comes cleansing. That's where ubtan comes in. Ubtan isn't just one recipe, it's a whole family of them, all with the same spirit. Usually, it starts with gram flour or another ground lentil, which gives the paste a gentle grit. Turmeric almost always shows up, because it calms redness and gives skin a warm glow. Some families add sandalwood for scent, neem for its reputation, milk or yogurt for softness, and a little oil for extra comfort.

The paste gets mixed fresh before a bath. Rosewater or plain water turns the powders into something you can spread. This is where it becomes a ritual, not just a recipe. Ubtan goes on in slow circles. Arms, legs, face, and sometimes everywhere. It dries a bit, tightens, then you rub it off and rinse. Dust, sweat, and the week's dullness go with it. What's left? Softer skin, a hint of turmeric and sandalwood, and usually a calmer mood. Some people say it scrubs off more than just dead skin. Maybe that's not scientific, but it sure feels true.

For brides in India, Pakistan, and Bangladesh, this takes on greater significance. The haldi ceremony, where loved ones apply a special turmeric-rich ubtan before the wedding, is a celebration of both beauty and blessing. Laughter, teasing, and bright yellow hands everywhere. It is skincare, yes, but it is also a way of saying, "We surround you with love as you step into a new life." Much like the practice of covering a bride in henna in Middle Eastern weddings, the haldi ritual underscores a universal theme: love and unity enveloping the bride as she embarks on a new journey.

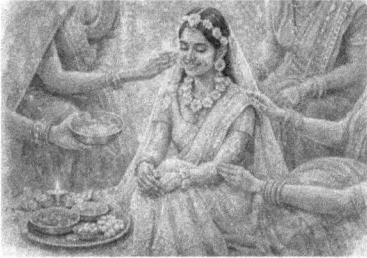

Soap wasn't always around, and when it was, it wasn't always gentle. So, people used what they had, which was clays and bath powders. Multani mitti, a pale clay, is still used as a face mask to soak up oil and calm skin. Teenagers mix it with water when they get a breakout, just like their parents did. For hair, there was reetha (soapnut) and shikakai, both plant cleansers that got the job done without stripping your hair. It's interesting to think that you can wash your hair with fruit or clean your face with clay from the ground.

Cleanliness can come from the same place as your food.

Fragrance weaves through South Asian beauty in its own delicate way. Instead of spray perfumes, traditional scents often arrive as attars, concentrated oils distilled from flowers, wood, or spices. In certain cities, perfumers have spent generations capturing the essence of jasmine, rose, vetiver, and even the smell of the first monsoon rain falling on dry earth. A tiny drop behind the ears, at the wrists, or in the hair is enough. The oil warms on the skin and releases a soft, intimate scent that does not shout; it lingers. Sandalwood oil is another quiet luxury. Smoothed on the skin in the heat of summer, it feels cooling, grounded, and deeply comforting. These scents become part of a person's identity. People remember them the way they remember a voice.

Bathing itself carries a spiritual tone in many homes. A morning snān is seen as preparation not just for the day but for prayer, for work, for showing up in the world clean in every sense. In rural areas, bathing in rivers or under an open sky can feel less like a task and more like a conversation with nature. Rough washcloths, dried gourds turned into scrubbers, and brisk rubbing bring blood to the surface, leaving the skin tingling. A splash of rosewater afterward or a thin streak of sandalwood paste on the forehead helps the body stay cool and lightly perfumed, which matters in climates where heat is a daily companion.

Men's grooming has its own rich story here, though it often overlaps with women's routines. The concept of "champi," a vigorous head massage, is famous enough that it eventually gave English the word "shampoo." In bustling old cities, barbers would offer a quick champi on the street, kneading oils into the scalp with practiced intensity. Travelers were astonished at how revived they felt afterward. Over time, the word that once referred to the massage itself came to mean the cleansing step we all know. Yet in many barbershops, the original practice remains. After a haircut, a man may lean back for a brief head or face massage, walking out with hair trimmed and stress dialed down a notch.

Another old skill, threading, has surged in popularity far beyond its origins. Using a simple twisted cotton thread, practitioners pluck hair with swift precision from brows, upper lips, and other areas. It is efficient, tidy, and requires no chemicals. For centuries, it was part of everyday grooming in South Asia and the Middle East. Now it is a sought-after technique in malls and salons around the world.

Modern Trends and Adaptations

Let's take, for example, the turmeric face mask. For many South Asians, it was always just there, used for weddings, special days, or as a weekly treat. For others, the idea of putting yellow spice on your face sounded odd. But as people heard about turmeric's benefits, curiosity turned into a trend. Suddenly, social media was full of people mixing turmeric with yogurt or honey in their bathrooms. Some brands promised miracles. But at the heart of it, this was just a kitchen ingredient that had worked for generations, finally getting noticed.

Hair oiling took a similar journey. For a while, some younger people called it old-fashioned and preferred lots of products instead. Then the conversation changed. People started caring about scalp health and simple routines. Suddenly, warming oil and massaging it in sounded smart, not outdated. Influencers with South Asian roots shared their oil routines, and people noticed how healthy their hair looked. Curly hair communities picked it up too. The hashtag grew, brands jumped in, and everyone had advice. Underneath it all, there was a simple truth: this old habit was right all along.

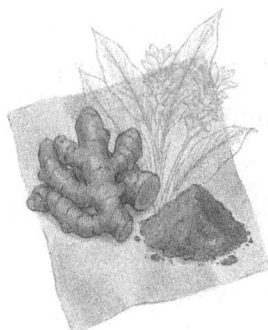

Inside South Asia, things go both ways now. In a bathroom in Mumbai or Karachi, you might see a neem face wash next to a Korean sheet mask and European sunscreen. Local brands know this. Their message is simple: we took what your family used and made it fit your schedule. Tradition just comes in new packaging now. Picture a college student in Delhi, multitasking between classes, who starts the day with a neem wash, incorporates a K-beauty toner in the afternoon, and finishes with a European moisturizer at night. This everyday scene illustrates the cultural fusion that defines modern beauty routines, merging ancestral practices with global innovations.

Social media made it easier for men to say they care about their skin and scent. Barbers who used to just cut hair and shave now offer facials with sandalwood or turmeric, shoulder massages with oils, and even advice on which attar goes with your cologne. The old champi is still there, but now it sits next to sheet masks and serums. The point is simple: taking care of yourself isn't vanity. It's just maintenance for a busy life.

As people talk more about waste and sustainability, old South Asian solutions are coming back. Soapnuts for laundry and hair, reusable cloths, and shampoo bars made from clay and oil—these old ideas fit right in with new eco-friendly values. People tired of long ingredient lists and plastic bottles like the idea of washing with a handful of nuts or a simple bar. In a way, the world is just catching up to what many South Asian homes never stopped doing. Consider this: When was the last time you treated grooming as recovery, not just routine? By embracing these sustainable practices, men can find both an eco-friendly and refreshing approach to self-care.

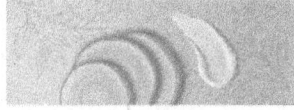

Makeup tells its own story. Kajal, the traditional black liner, was originally made at home from soot and oils. This simple mixture was said to protect the eyes from the harsh sun and ward off evil spirits, imparting both decorative and protective qualities. Today, kajal comes in pencils and twist-up sticks, sold everywhere as the secret to a smoky look. Inside South Asia, makeup choices have exploded, with more shades and styles than ever. However, small things like a bindi or a line of vermilion still hold deeper meanings beyond mere aesthetics. A person's routine can mix new products, old symbols, and personal style all at once.

Ayurvedic spa treatments are another example. People abroad book oil pours or four-hand massages, hoping for deep relaxation. This outside interest has made locals look again at old therapies. Now, weekend retreats and wellness centers in India offer these treatments to people who once thought they were just for older generations. A young professional might even save up for a traditional detox. Heritage isn't just respected now—it's something to aim for.

With all the change, at the core of South Asian beauty is a simple idea: use what's close to the earth, pay attention, and remember that balance matters more than perfection. You see it in a grandmother mixing ubtan by hand, trusting her touch. You see it in a teenager who finds the same mask online and realizes her new trend is her family's old way.

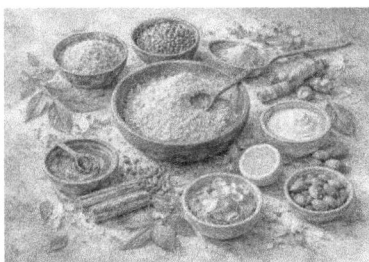

DIY Ubtan: A Traditional Glow Mask

One of the easiest ways to try this for yourself is to make a basic ubtan at home. No special store, no fancy tools. Just a few ingredients and a bit of time.

Here's how to do it:

•1. Gather the ingredients.

Start with two tablespoons of gram flour. Add a teaspoon of turmeric. Mix in a tablespoon of plain yogurt for moisture and a teaspoon of honey to help your skin stay hydrated. If you have sandalwood powder, add a pinch. It's optional, but it smells great and feels calming.

•2. Mix into a paste.

Add your liquid slowly. Rosewater is traditional and feels fancy, but milk or water works too. Stir until it's smooth and spreadable—

like cake batter. Thick enough to stay on your skin, soft enough to move under your fingers.

·3. Apply gently.

On clean skin, spread the paste in gentle circles over your face or body. Take your time. Notice the grainy flour and the cool yogurt. Avoid your eyes— turmeric stings if it comes into contact.

4. Let it set.

Let the ubtan sit until it's partly dry—five to ten minutes for your face, a bit longer for your body. Don't let it crack. You want it just firm enough to feel like it's done its job.

5. Rinse and massage off.

Wet your hands and gently re-moisten the mask, then use small circles to loosen and rinse it off. This gives you a little extra exfoliation. If your skin is very light, you might see a yellow tint, but it fades. Some people even leave it a bit longer for extra turmeric benefits.

6. Moisturize.

Pat your skin dry. If it needs more comfort, rub in a few drops of coconut or almond oil. Usually, the yogurt and honey have already left your skin soft.

Check your skin after. It usually feels smoother, looks brighter, and smells earthy. That's the obvious result. But there's something else, too. For a few minutes, you joined a ritual that's been around for generations.

You can keep this recipe simple or use it as a base. If you break out easily, add a pinch of neem powder. If your skin is dry, try mashed banana for more moisture. Ubtan is flexible, much like the culture it comes from. The only rule? Use it with care. Not rushed. Not as a chore. Just as a small, intentional act of looking after yourself.

When you rinse off the mask, hands stained gold, you're having a "mask day" and joining a long line of people who believed beauty and well-being start with simple things, gentle touch, and a little time for yourself. That's the best glow.

CHAPTER 2

East Asia – Serenity, Steam, and Skincare Science

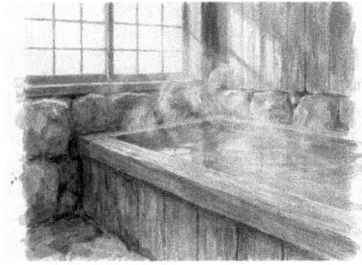

Across East Asia, beauty isn't something you rush through. It's a ritual, sometimes shared with others, sometimes done alone in front of the mirror, but always intentional. Whether it's soaking in a hot spring, layering on skincare, or rinsing hair with rice water, the focus is the same: take your time, work with your body, and let nature help you out.

Traditional Rituals and Timeless Techniques

East Asia holds a wide range of cultures, but many of their beauty customs seem to nod to one another. Japan's measured onsen rituals, Korea's vigorous jjimjilbang scrubs, China's herbal wisdom and rice water rinses. All are built on a few simple ideas: cleanse deeply, restore balance, and treat beauty as something that is grown, not painted on.

Take the Japanese onsen. You clean yourself first, then get into the hot spring once you're sure you're spotless. The water is full of minerals people say help with sore joints and irritated skin. It's more than hygiene. It's about taking care of yourself, inside and out.

You relax, your muscles let go, and even the air seems quieter. In winter, they'll toss citrus fruits in the water for a little luck and a fresh scent.

Korean jjimjilbangs are a whole different vibe. Here, getting clean is serious business. After soaking, you get scrubbed down with rough mitts until you see dead skin roll off. It's a little awkward at first, but the feeling afterward of smooth skin and a sense of starting fresh, is worth it.

After the scrub, you put on comfy clothes and hang out with friends or family in warm rooms. People nap, drink tea, snack, and move between saunas and cool spaces. It's part bathhouse, part living room. That same thoroughness is in Korean skincare too. The double cleanse which is oil first, then foam, gives your face a gentle but deep clean. No harsh stuff, just steady care.

China has its own take, with a big focus on herbal baths and remedies. The idea is simple: what you eat and drink shows up on your skin, so inside and outside care go together. One standout? Rice water for hair. Women have used the leftover water from rinsing rice to wash their hair for generations. The result is strong, shiny hair which surprised a lot of people who thought you needed fancy products.

You don't need a lab report to get it. Rice water has starches and nutrients that make hair smoother and less likely to break. Running a comb through rinsed hair each morning becomes its own kind of meditation. A small habit that quietly protects.

Tea isn't just for drinking. In East Asia, it ends up in bathwater and skincare too. Green tea baths in Japan add antioxidants and a fresh scent. Homemade masks in China and Korea often use cooled tea. Broths, soups, and teas have been part of beauty routines for generations, long before wellness trends made them popular.

Another big idea: good circulation shows on your face. Gua sha is a classic example. It started as a way to scrape the body and boost energy, but for beauty, it's gentler. You use a smooth stone with oil to massage your face and neck, which helps with puffiness and blood flow. Jade rollers do something similar. Rolling a cool stone over your skin helps relax muscles and lift your mood.

These tools have traveled far, but at their core they still represent a simple idea: touch heals. A slow massage while cleansing or moisturizing, whether in Tokyo, Seoul, or Beijing, is not a gimmick. It is built on an understanding that the face is not a separate object. It is connected to muscles, lymph, and emotion, and they all respond to kind attention.

There's a long history in East Asia of wanting clear, even skin. Sometimes that meant a preference for very pale skin, as a sign you didn't work outside. That led to some odd beauty tricks. Japanese courtesans used masks made from sanitized nightingale droppings to refine their skin. In China, people swallowed ground pearls or used them as a paste for radiance. These sound wild now, but they came from a deep wish for smooth, glowing skin.

Now, the focus is less about being super pale and more about having clear, glowing skin. This is what Koreans call 'glass skin.' It's about keeping your skin hydrated, protecting it from the sun, and sticking to a daily routine. Sunscreen, hats, and taking care of your skin barrier aren't about looks. They're about prevention. It's daily self-care that pays off.

Modern Innovations and Viral Trends

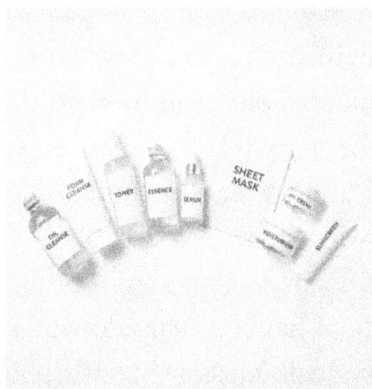

Korean beauty kicked things off with its multi-step routines. People joke about the '10-step routine,' and about the approach. Instead of scrubbing hard and slapping on one cream, you break it down: oil cleanse, foam cleanse, toner, essence, serum, sheet mask, eye cream, moisturizer, sunscreen. You can use a lot of products or just a few, but the idea is the same: layer hydration, add nourishment, and make skincare something you enjoy.

The world initially raised an eyebrow. Then people tried a single sheet mask and felt how plump and calm their face looked afterward.

Curious minds started playing with snail mucin essences, rice bran washes, and ginseng serums. Before long, drugstore aisles in cities far from Seoul were stocked with products inspired by ingredients from East Asia.

Japanese beauty went another way. Instead of adding more steps, it focused on fewer and simpler products. Cleansing oils that remove makeup without drying you out. Light lotions that hydrate without stinging. Moisturizers that help your skin do its job. And sunscreens that feel good and don't leave a white cast. When products feel this nice, using them every day is easy.

There's also *jamsu*, where you set your makeup with powder and dunk your face in cold water. It looks strange, but people say it helps makeup last. And then there's slugging. That is putting ointment over your skincare at night to lock in moisture. These trends took off online because they work for a lot of people.

China's influence is growing fast too. Herbal skincare went viral, and suddenly, young people who used to ignore traditional remedies are reaching for ginseng, lotus, and mushroom serums. Gua sha tools are everywhere now, not just in medicine cabinets. Meanwhile, some in

Japan started talking about 'skin fasting'—taking a break from heavy routines to let your skin reset.

Men are part of this trend too. K-Pop and J-Pop stars showed that taking care of your skin isn't just for women. Now, lots of men in Seoul, Tokyo, and Shanghai use toner, essence, and sunscreen every day. The message is simple: skin is skin, and everyone benefits from taking care of it.

The biggest change? Gentleness and prevention matter more now. Harsh scrubs and stinging toners are out. Instead, people use gentle cleansers, calming toners, hydrating essences, and sunscreens they actually like. The goal is to protect your skin, not punish it. When you treat skincare like brushing your teeth, it's something you do every day without drama.

Gua Sha Facial Massage: Ancient Tool, Modern Glow

If you want to invite a bit of East Asian ritual into your own routine, a simple gua sha face massage is a beautiful place to start. It is low effort, soothing, and all you really need is a smooth stone tool and a few drops of oil.

Here's how to do it:

1. Prepare your skin.

Start with a freshly cleansed face. Press a few drops of facial oil or a nourishing serum onto your skin so the tool can glide easily. Jojoba, sweet almond, or any comfortable face oil will do. Think of this step as setting the stage. You are giving your skin slip, comfort, and a little extra nourishment.

2. Sweep along the jawline.

Hold the tool almost flat against your skin, at about a fifteen-degree angle. Place it at the center of your chin and slowly sweep along the jaw toward your ear. Use gentle, steady pressure that moves the skin slightly rather than just skimming the surface. Repeat this four or five times on one side, then move to the other. You may notice that with each stroke, your jaw feels a bit less tight.

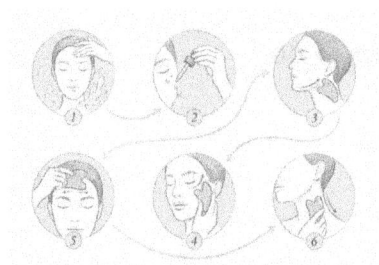

3.   Glide over the cheeks.

Next, position the tool beside your nose and sweep it outward over your cheekbone toward the temple. Follow the natural shape of your face. This motion can help move fluid away from the center and give the cheeks a slight lift. A few passes on each side are enough. Feel the stress melt a little as you go. You are not just shaping your face. You are easing muscles that have been clenching through conversations, emails, and small frustrations.

4. Brighten the under-eye area.

Using the softest pressure and the curved edge of the tool, start at the inner corner under the eye and sweep toward the outer corner. This area is delicate, so think feather touch. Two or three light strokes on each side can help morning puffiness settle down. It is less about sculpting and more about coaxing fluid gently where it needs to go.

5. Soften brow and forehead tension.

Place the tool at the inner end of your eyebrow and move it along the brow bone toward the temple. Many people are surprised by how good this feels the first time. Screen time and frowning leave a lot of tension here. Then move to the forehead. Begin between the brows and sweep upward toward the hairline. Work across the forehead in sections. With each stroke, imagine you are smoothing out not just lines, but thoughts that have been looping all day.

6. Finish with the neck.

Do not forget the neck. Starting just behind the ear, sweep the tool down along the side of the neck toward the collarbone. This helps fluid move gently where your body already knows how to handle it. You can also massage upward along the back and sides of the neck to ease tight muscles, avoiding direct pressure on the throat. A few slow sweeps are plenty.

7. Clean and notice.

Rinse or wipe your gua sha tool and let it dry. Then, simply feel your face with your hands. It will likely feel warmer, more awake, and oddly lighter. You can add a final layer of moisturizer if you like, although the oil you used often provides enough comfort.

The whole ritual can be done in five minutes or stretched longer on nights when you need extra unwinding. Some people keep their stone in the fridge for a cool, refreshing sensation in the morning. Over time, many notice less puffiness, a more relaxed expression, and a small pocket of calm built into their day.

Most of all, gua sha reminds you of something easy to forget. Your face is not simply something the world looks at. It is part of your body that deserves gentle, intentional touch. When you glide that stone along your skin, you are participating in a practice that has traveled quietly from ancient households to modern bathrooms. Old wisdom, new context. A small daily gesture that says, without many words, "I am worth a few minutes of my own careful attention."

CHAPTER 3

Southeast Asia – Tropical Traditions and Spice-Infused Beauty

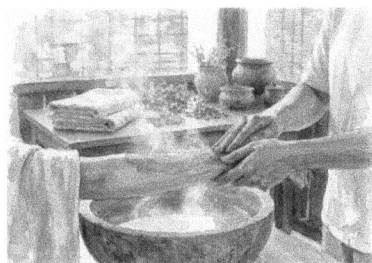

In Bali, morning light slips through bamboo as a bride sits very still. Her soft gold skin shines beneath a turmeric, rice, and jasmine oil mixture lovingly smoothed onto it. In a Thai village, herbal steam rises from clay pots filled with lemongrass, ginger, and kaffir lime. A new mother inhales the steam while the older women speak in low voices nearby. And, on a different island, coconut palms tilt over a small courtyard where a grandmother works oil into a child's scalp. She has the easy surety of someone who's done this more times than she could count.

Traditional Practices: Spice, Herb, and Harmony

This part of the world is so lush, it almost feels unreal. It seems like everywhere you look you see rainforests, rice fields, spice gardens, and fruit. Of course, people here used what was right in front of them. Roots, barks, flowers, leaves, rice, and coconut. Basically, nature stocked their bathroom shelves for them.

What stands out about Southeast Asian rituals is how they mix everything. A scrub isn't just about soft skin. A bath isn't just about getting clean. Beauty, health, and even a little bit of soul care all happens at once. Some of these started as royal secrets, others in regular kitchens. Now, you'll find them everywhere from fancy spas to your neighbor's bathroom.

Take the Javanese lulur.

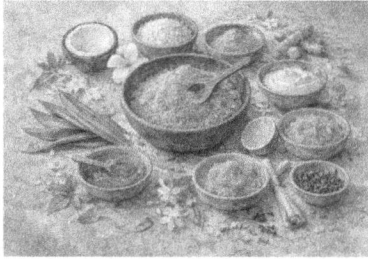

Lulur began as a royal pre-wedding ritual in Java, designed to prepare the bride's skin and spirit for her new life. The word itself suggests coating and massaging, which is precisely what happens. A paste is made from ground rice, turmeric, sandalwood, and other local herbs like pandan and candlenut, mixed with water or milk until it becomes a fragrant, grainy cream.

The paste is massaged all over the body. At first, it feels gritty and slightly cool. As hands move in slow circles, warmth rises in the skin, and the spices begin to release their scent. When the scrub is rinsed off, the skin is smoothed, gently polished, and faintly stained gold from the turmeric. That's only the first act.

Often, yogurt or milk is then smoothed over the freshly scrubbed skin, soaking in easily and leaving a soft, velvety finish. A floral bath may follow: warm water scattered with jasmine, rose petals, and ylang-ylang blossoms. You can imagine the scene. Grit giving way to cream. Earthy spice giving way to sweet flowers. A bride stepping out not just with glowing skin, but with a quieter heart.

Spas in Bali and Java offer lulur as a must-try treatment. You can even buy pre-mixed lulur powder and keep it in your bathroom for a weekly pick-me-up. What used to be a big deal for brides is now just a way to say, 'I deserve to feel special today.'

Thailand has its own kind of magic.

Herbal compresses, known locally as luk pra kob, look simple at first glance. Bundles of cotton stuffed with chopped herbs: lemongrass, kaffir lime peel, turmeric, ginger, tamarind leaves, sometimes camphor. These bundles are steamed until piping hot and then pressed, rolled, and patted over the body in a rhythmic massage.

People have used these for ages to relieve sore muscles and support recovery after childbirth. The heat gets right into your muscles. The herbs do their thing, and you can feel your back loosen up, your shoulders relax, and your breathing slow down. You feel looked after. You feel like someone's got your back.

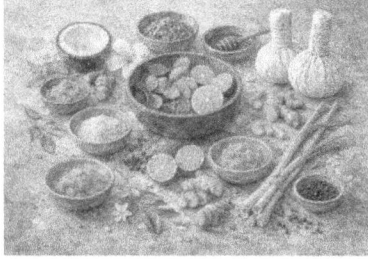

Afterward, your skin carries a delicate scent of spices and citrus. In some traditions, the heat of the compress is balanced with a bath in cooler water scented with flowers like jasmine or chrysanthemum. Hot and cool. Stimulation and calm. The same balance that keeps the body calm also keeps the complexion happy.

Then there is *thanaka* in Myanmar.

In Myanmar, you'll see people with pale yellow designs on their cheeks. These designs are big circles, stripes, or leaf patterns. That's thanaka, made by grinding tree bark on a stone. It keeps skin calm, works as a natural sunscreen, and helps with oily skin and breakouts. But it's more than that. Moms teach their kids how to use it. Friends draw patterns on each other's faces. It's skincare, sun care, and a bit of cultural pride. Even with new creams available, many people still prefer to grind the bark fresh every day.

In the Philippines, the hero is the coconut.

Coconut oil, called lana in many regions, is everywhere. Historically, it moisturized skin, treated minor irritations, and conditioned hair. Many Filipinos grew up with memories of "hilot," a traditional massage using warm coconut oil, given by a parent or local healer. After a bath, a child might be laid on a mat and gently kneaded from head to toe until the day's tension melted away.

Hair care? Same story. Coconut oil goes into hair to make it stronger, shinier, and to keep away lice or dryness. Some people save rice water from cooking and use it as a face toner. Milk baths, just coconut or goat's milk in water, make your skin feel soft and special. Aloe vera grows in pots outside, ready to be split open and used on burns, itchy scalps, or weak hair. It's all simple, direct, and it works.

Vietnam adds another layer of herbal creativity.

Herbs and rice wine have long been combined for both internal tonics and external rubs. After childbirth or hard labor, women might use herb-infused rice wine as a brisk body rub to warm and stimulate circulation. Diluted, similar concoctions can be patted onto the skin to invigorate.

And let's not forget leaf baths. People simmer lemongrass, ginger, basil, or whatever's on hand, then pour that fragrant water into the bath or use it for a steamy rinse. If you walk past a courtyard that smells like lemongrass, someone's probably treating themselves to a special bath. It's a total reset for your senses.

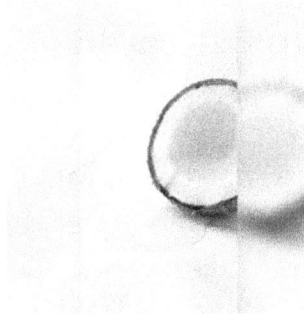

Hair traditions across Southeast Asia share this same imagination—coconut milk or aloe masks in Malaysia and Indonesia. Smoke perfumes the hair in certain Javanese rituals, as fragrant resins and woods are burned and the hair is exposed to the curling smoke. The result is hair that smells faintly of incense and flowers, with the bonus of the smoke's antimicrobial qualities.

Many of these rituals happen at big life moments. In Malaysia, new moms receive belly binding, herbal baths, scrubs, and hot-stone massages to help them recover. In Bali or Thailand, weddings bring together a group of aunties, cousins, and friends to scrub, bathe, and dress the bride. There's laughter, advice, and the smell of herbs. Here, beauty is about your community showing up for you when life is changing.

Modern Blends and Revival

Just like everywhere else, Southeast Asia's old rituals are changing and spreading. Spas all over the world offer 'Balinese body polish' or 'Thai herbal therapy,' often copying the real thing.

At the same time, local brands are updating their beauty routines. They're using the same heritage ingredients like turmeric, rice, tamarind, pandan, hibiscus, ginger, lemongrass, galangal, and kaffir lime. You'll also find them in cleansers, toners, scrubs, and masks with modern packaging.

Holistic thinking remains strong. A turmeric body scrub sits on the same mental shelf as a turmeric-and-tamarind tonic. If you drink well, you glow. If you scrub well, you sleep better. Health and beauty are not separate lanes.

Social media turned a lot of these old habits into global 'hacks.' Coconut oil suddenly became the go-to for hair, body, and even makeup removal.

Tropical fruits and kitchen staples got their moment, too. People used to mash up papaya to soften rough skin and exfoliate, thanks to the natural enzymes. Now, you'll find papaya enzymes in bottles of cleanser and peel. Tamarind pulp, once used in Thai and Malay baths for brighter skin, is now in brightening products. Overripe bananas mixed with coconut milk and honey were the original hair mask and now there are banana conditioners everywhere. The internet made everyone try putting just about anything on their face, so companies started making neater, less messy versions.

In cities like Manila, Bangkok, or Jakarta, men's barbershops mix global trends with local touches. Aftershaves might smell like calamansi (a small, tart local citrus fruit), and pomades might use coconut oil. Some guys go for old-school hair oils that look like something their granddad used, but now they feel cool again. Others just add a herbal compress or a spa day to deal with stress. The idea that self-care is just for women is fading fast. The attitude here is simple: if it helps you feel better, why not?

Fragrance is another gift from Southeast Asia. Agarwood, or *oud*, is one of the most famous. Resins from trees in Vietnam, Laos, and nearby areas end up in luxury perfumes around the world. Agarwood was once burned in ceremonies or used to scent clothes. Now, it's in expensive perfumes. Small perfumers in Bali, Bangkok, and elsewhere blend ylang-ylang, champaka, frangipani, local spices, and resins. The result is scents that remind you of warm nights and temple incense. This is something locals and visitors both want to take home.

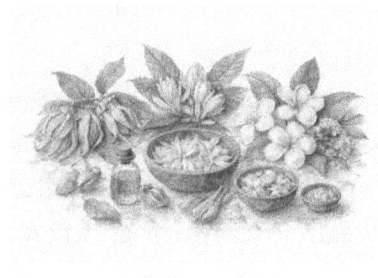

People are also thinking more about the environment. A lot of folks are going back to old, low-waste habits. Natural luffa gourds are making a comeback instead of plastic shower puffs. Herb gardens with pandan, lemongrass, and basil are popping up on balconies for homemade bath infusions. Workshops teach you how to make your own spice scrubs or coconut oil.

Of course, not everyone wants to DIY everything. That's why stores are now full of greener options: shampoo bars with local herbs, reef-safe sunscreen made from island ingredients, packaging with batik prints or local art. So, you can take care of yourself and still respect your roots and the environment.

Mixing routines are normal now. Someone in Thailand might use Korean skincare most days but still grab their mom's turmeric scrub on the weekend. In the Philippines, you might see Japanese shampoo, French conditioner, and then a rinse with gugo bark water for strong hair. Travelers might keep a Western serum next to a homemade herbal compress. The point? Pick what works for you.

Modern beauty here isn't about choosing just one way. It's about making your own routine from lots of different pieces. If you think about it, that's what these traditions have always been about anyway.

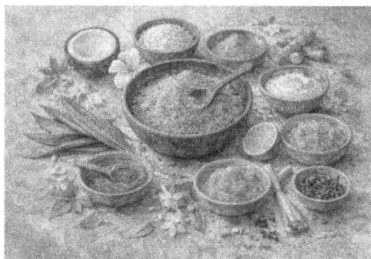

Tropical Body Scrub: A Lulur-Inspired Home Ritual

You don't need a plane ticket or a fancy spa to get a taste of Southeast Asian luxury. Turn your shower into a mini retreat with a lulur-inspired body scrub using what you already have in your kitchen. It's simple, it feels great, and it's a good reminder to slow down and take care of yourself.

What you'll need

2 tablespoons turmeric powder

4 tablespoons rice flour (or finely ground oats)

2 tablespoons brown sugar

Zest of 1 lime or lemon

3–4 tablespoons milk, yogurt, or coconut milk

Turmeric gives warmth and a little glow. Rice flour or oats scrub gently. Brown sugar polishes and keeps things moist. Citrus zest wakes up your senses. Milk or coconut milk brings it all together into a creamy, soothing paste.

Mix the scrub

Mix the turmeric, rice flour, and brown sugar in a bowl. Add the lime or lemon zest and stir again. Pour in your liquid a little at a time until it's thick and spreadable. You want it to stick to your skin but still be easy to move around. If you're not sure, aim for something like loose cookie dough and not runny batter.

Apply with intention

Step into the shower, turn off the water for a bit, and give yourself some space. Grab a handful of scrub and start massaging it onto your skin in circles. Begin at your ankles and work your way up.

This is where the ritual lives.

Feel the grains working to smooth your skin. Notice the warmth from the turmeric, the fresh citrus scent, and the sweetness from the sugar. Use enough pressure to wake up your skin, but don't go overboard. Focus on rough spots, such as elbows, knees, and heels. Let your mind follow your hands. This isn't just about getting clean. It's a way of telling yourself, 'My body deserves some care.'

Let it rest for a moment.

If you have a few minutes, just pause with the scrub still on your skin. Lean against the wall, take a breath, and let the ingredients do their thing. The turmeric calms, the milk or coconut milk softens, and the scent fills the air. For a moment, your bathroom isn't just a bathroom. It's your own private spa.

Rinse away what you no longer need.

Turn the water back on and rinse well. Use your hands to help the scrub wash away, and watch the golden swirls go down the drain. If your skin looks a little yellow (especially if you're fair), just use some gentle soap and a washcloth, or let it fade naturally.

Seal in the softness.

Pat yourself dry. Run your hands over your arms and legs. They'll feel smoother, more awake, and lightly scented. If you want, finish with a bit of body oil or lotion. Coconut oil with a drop of jasmine or ylang-ylang is a nice nod to the traditional lulur finish.

What you just did is both a recipe and a little piece of a tradition that used to be for queens and brides, now made for your regular Tuesday. You took simple things from your kitchen and turned them into a way to show your body some respect.

In Southeast Asia, these rituals have always been about a combination of things. They help people through big changes, honor new moms, prepare brides, and give everyone a chance to look and feel new again. When you do even a small part of that at home, you're joining in that same story, even if just for a moment.

And that, as much as the softness of your skin afterward, is the true blessing.

CHAPTER 4

North Africa and the Middle East – Hammams and Sacred Scents

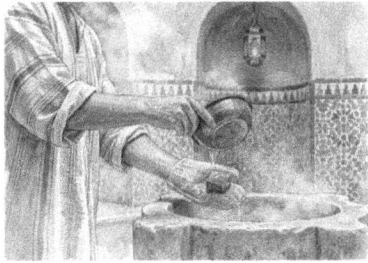

Step into a hammam in Marrakech, and you'll find steam, laughter, and the sharp scent of black soap. Women are scrubbing each other's backs and trading stories. They are letting go of the week's stress and bonding at the same time. A soap seller in Damascus stacks green bars of olive and laurel, and a customer breathes in the clean scent, maybe thinking of home. A mother in Dubai dabs white musk behind her daughter's ears after a bath, just like her own mother did. They're small acts of care passed down through generations.

In North Africa and the Middle East, getting clean is more than washing off dirt. It's about faith, hospitality, scent, and the fundamental need to feel like yourself again.

Traditional Rituals: Bathing, Scrubbing, Scenting

A lot of what the world considers ritual bathing began here. The hammam, black soap, clay, oils—these were perfected in this region and shared with the world, one generation at a time.

A classic Moroccan hammam is simple but powerful. You start in the heat, letting your body relax and your pores open. Then you smooth on black soap, a thick, dark soap made from olives. It doesn't foam very much. It just softens your skin and helps you let go of whatever the week has left behind.

After a few minutes, you rinse. Then the transformation begins.

Next comes the kessa glove. It's a rough mitt for scrubbing. You work it over your arms, shoulders, stomach, and legs. Suddenly, you see gray rolls of dead skin. It's a little gross and a little funny. Moroccan women say you're not really clean until you see those "snakes" of skin. For them, this deep scrub is just regular upkeep, like vacuuming. It's intense, but it wakes you up. Your skin feels alive.

After scrubbing, you might use a clay mask called rhassoul from the Atlas Mountains, mixed with water or rosewater. You spread it on and wait. Maybe someone massages your scalp, or perhaps you just listen to the sounds around you. When you rinse it all off, your skin feels almost new.

Afterward, you step into cooler air and smooth on a bit of argan oil or olive oil. Just a thin layer does the trick. The oil soaks in fast, leaving your skin soft and a little shiny. Then you rest and wrap up in a towel, sip some mint tea, and let your body cool down. It's a reset from heavy to light.

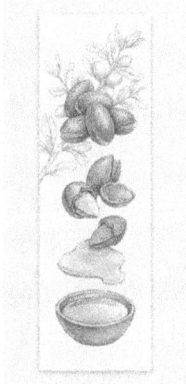

This way of bathing isn't just Moroccan. Turkish hammams, Persian and

Egyptian bathhouses, they all share the same spirit. These places are about more than getting clean. They're where people talk, laugh, share news, and get ready for big moments like weddings. Cleanliness here is about your body and your mood.

Fragrance holds its own sacred place.

For many, a bath isn't finished until you add scent. Perfume oils, called attars, are pressed onto your wrists or behind your ears. White musk is a favorite because it smells clean and soft. It's a private scent, close to the skin, more for you than anyone else.

Oud is another key scent. People burn it as incense and wave their clothes through the smoke so the smell sticks. Guests are often offered the burner as a way to say, 'You're welcome here.' Homes and hotels use it too. It's as if they are saying "we want you to feel good here."

Kohl is another thread that began long ago and shows no sign of fading.

Lining your eyes with dark kohl goes way back to ancient Egypt. It was made from minerals or soot and used by everyone, men and women, to protect their eyes from the sun and from bad luck. Today, the formulas are safer, but the look is the same: bold lines, bigger eyes. When you see dramatic 'Arab eyes,' you're seeing a tradition that's thousands of years old. After you look at the eyes, you'll naturally look at the skin, and then hair.

Daily skin and hair care here grew out of the climate. Dry air and intense sun mean you need gentle cleansing and lots of moisture. Olive oil soaps were the answer—simple bars that clean without drying you out. Aleppo soap is the classic example, used for both the body and hair, and it inspired many soaps that followed.

People also used simple minerals. Alum stones worked as a natural deodorant and to calm shaving cuts. Sugar, boiled with lemon and water became halawa. This is the sticky paste for hair removal. If you grew up here, you probably remember sitting in a warm kitchen while your mom or aunt spread the sugar on your skin and flicked it off. Painful? Yes. But also a bonding moment. And it works.

Henna is both decoration and care. The leaves are ground and mixed into a paste that stains your skin with detailed designs for weeks. Before weddings and festivals, hands and feet are covered in patterns that look like lace. The same plant, used on hair, adds a reddish tint and makes it stronger and softer. This one plant has many uses and deep meaning.

Fragrance is part of hospitality, too. Guests are offered tea or coffee, but also scent. Wafts of oud smoke drifting their way, or a bottle of perfume oil passed around. Sharing scent is just another way of saying, 'We're glad you're here. Take something good with you.'

Contemporary Trends: Revival and Reinvention

For years, mainstream beauty focused on other places. Now, people are finally paying attention to what North Africa and the Middle East have always done as real, effective care.

Take argan oil. Berber women in Morocco have used it for generations to soften skin and hair and even to cook. Eventually, the rest of the world caught on. Now it's in shampoos, serums, and face oils everywhere because it softens without leaving a greasy residue. Its popularity also sparked new conversations about fair trade and ensuring the women who make it get their share. Beauty and ethics can go together.

Rosewater and orange blossom water took a similar route. They were once found mainly in Middle Eastern grocery stores, as desserts or to soothe skin. Now, you'll find them in beauty aisles everywhere. People spray rosewater to refresh makeup or just feel better during a long day. What seems new is old. They are just in new packaging.

Other kitchen staples such as black seed oil, pomegranate, dates, and coffee, are now also in modern beauty products. Seeds, fruits, and beans that have been long used at home are finally getting their moment in moisturizers and scrubs. Here, the line between kitchen and bathroom has always been thin. The rest of the world is just catching up.

Local entrepreneurs and influencers are sharing these traditions in new ways. Beauty founders from Iraq, the Gulf, North Africa, and the Levant are building brands that celebrate bold brows, dramatic lashes, strong scents, and glowing skin. They talk openly about the routines they learned from their family. Perfume houses in the region create modern scents that still honor oud, rose, and musk, and they teach people how to layer and create their own blends.

Online, old tools are making a comeback. Natural tooth sticks are now called eco-friendly toothbrushes. Alum stones are back as crystal deodorants. Sugaring, once something you did at home, is now offered in fancy studios as a gentler alternative to waxing. These practices never really went away.

Traditional barbers still do close shaves and head massages, but now you'll also find fades, beard shaping, and a lineup of colognes. Men here have always worn fragrance proudly—rose, oud, amber, not just citrus. As the world moves past strict scent rules, unisex and layered fragrances are becoming normalized.

At home, younger people mix old and new without a second thought. Someone might use a fancy European cream after rinsing with rosewater; their grandmother swears by it. One week, it's a modern spa and the next, a traditional hammam. Maybe a Korean sheet mask one day, a yogurt-and-honey mask from mom the next. This isn't confusion. You can honor your roots and still enjoy what's out there.

There's a new sense of pride, too. "This is where I come from, and I think it's beautiful." is in style. What used to feel 'too traditional' is now shared openly. Tutorials like videos on kohl, of home hammam routines, and photos of hennaed hands before weddings are more normalized.

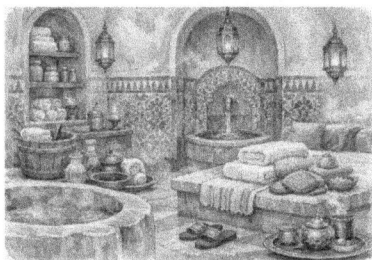

At-Home Hammam: A Weekly Reset

Create your own hammam-inspired ritual. This is your weekly reset and a way to get an even deeper clean.

1. Warm and soften

Start by taking a hot shower or bath and let the steam build. Breathe slowly, let the heat relax your muscles and your mind. Next, add a few drops of eucalyptus or mint oil to the shower wall or a bowl of hot water. The scented steam changes everything.

Stay in this warmth for five to ten minutes, until you feel your skin and shoulders relax.

2. Coat with soap

Step out of the water but keep your skin wet. If you have Moroccan black soap, use it. If not, pick a rich, gentle soap or an olive oil shower gel. You're not looking for foam, just a slippery layer.

Spread the soap all over and let it sit for a few minutes. Stand or sit quietly. Picture your tiredness loosening up, just like the dead skin.

3. Scrub with intention

Rinse off the soap with warm water. Put on a kessa glove or grab a textured washcloth. Start at your ankles and scrub in long, firm strokes—up your legs, over your hips, along your arms, and across your back and shoulders as far as you can reach.

You may start to see the dead skin come off. Do not be alarmed. This is precisely what you came for. Adjust the pressure so it feels strong but not punishing. Your skin will probably redden a bit. Your circulation is waking up.

If you are new to this level of exfoliation, go gently and skip very delicate areas. You are aiming for polished, not raw.

4. Optional clay mask

If you want to take it further, mix a simple body mask before you start: rhassoul clay with warm water, or even just plain yogurt with a drizzle of olive oil. After scrubbing and rinsing, smooth this mixture over your skin. Sit for five minutes, no more, and let it sit like a thin coat.

Rinse off completely. This step is like giving your fresh skin a little reward.

5. Cool down

Finish with a cool rinse if you can handle it. Even thirty seconds under cooler water wakes you up after all that heat. Your skin feels tighter, and your mind feels clearer.

Step out, wrap up in a towel or robe, and take a moment.

6. Oil and scent

While your skin is still damp, pour a little oil such as argan, olive, or almond, whatever you like, into your hands. Warm it up and massage it in slowly. Don't rush. Your skin will soak it up faster than usual after a scrub.

If you enjoy fragrance, dab a tiny amount of perfume oil on your wrists, behind your ears, or at the base of your throat. Choose something that feels clean and comforting to you. It does not have to be strong. This is more about how you feel than how others perceive you.

7. Rest, even briefly

If you can, give yourself 10 or 15 minutes of quiet afterward. Lie down, sip tea, or just sit and notice how your body feels. Heavy in a good way, warm and light at once.

You've drawn a line between this week and the next.

If you do this regularly, it stops being a treat and becomes a habit. It's a way of saying, 'I don't have to carry every bit of the week with me. I get to start fresh, in my own skin.'

CHAPTER 5

Sub-Saharan Africa – Roots of Radiance and Modern Revival

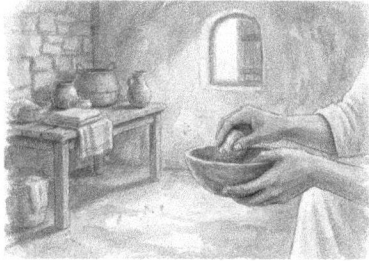

Imagine a young woman in Ghana making black soap under the hot sun. In Nigeria, you might see rows of bright sapo net sponges in the market, inviting you to try them for smoother skin. In Chad, a girl sits with friends, applying chebe powder and oil to her braids while they laugh about how much hair she has.

The beauty routines in Sub-Saharan Africa tend to be simple. People just use what's around them and press, grind, mix up whatever grows nearby.

Guess what? It works. The takeaway is that most of what you need nature already handed you.

Traditional Practices: Butters, Scrubs, and Protective Styles

Sub-Saharan Africa is massive, so forget about one-size-fits-all. The weather in Ghana is not even close to the dry heat in Kenya or the cool nights in Lesotho. But here's what you do see everywhere: skin that can handle sun and dust, hair that stays protected and healthy, and ingredients that are local legends.

Shea butter is probably the region's most famous export. People call it "women's gold" for a reason. Women's cooperatives gather the nuts, roast them, and knead them by hand into this rich, dense butter. In many West African homes, shea isn't a fancy treat. It's what you grab after a bath, what you rub into a baby's skin before heading out into the dry wind, what you use on cracked heels, chapped lips, or a stretching belly.

Shea butter is thick. If you grew up with it, you know the move: warm a little in your hands and press it in. Eventually, it's just part of your routine, part of your story. Ask an older woman with great skin what she uses, and she'll probably shrug and say, 'The same thing my mother used on me.'

African black soap is another quiet powerhouse.

In markets across Ghana, Nigeria, and other parts of West Africa, you can still find mounds of soft, dark soap sold in hand-shaped balls. It is usually made from plant ash, such as cocoa pod husks, plantain skins, or palm fronds, mixed with oils like palm kernel, coconut, or shea. The result is a crumbly, deep brown or black, earthy-smelling soap that foams into light, gentle lather.

Black soap seems to be a solution for just about everything for your face, body, and scalp. It gets rid of sweat and oil without leaving your skin dry, which matters when it's hot, and water isn't always easy to come by. Some say it helps with acne or evens out their skin tone. There's something satisfying about washing your face with soap made from ingredients you can picture growing nearby.

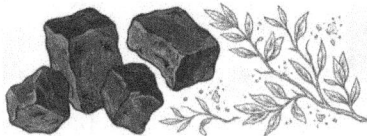

Exfoliation, too, has its own genius here.

Forget fancy brushes. Most families just use the African net sponge or "*sapo*" if you're in Ghana or Nigeria. It's a long, colorful strip of netting that looks basic but gets the job done. Once it's wet, it softens up but still scrubs like a champ. You can finally reach your back without twisting yourself into a pretzel. And it dries fast, so you don't get stuck with a musty, soggy mess like you do with a loofah.

For a lot of people, a shower just isn't a shower without a good scrub from the net sponge. Kids grow up with it. Adults rely on it to keep away rough patches and ingrown hairs. One sponge can last a year or more. Proof that the best ideas are usually the simplest.

Hair care might be where the region's creativity shines most.

Curly and coily hair needs moisture, patience, and protection. Many traditions revolve around those three needs. Braids, twists, cornrows, and other protective styles keep hair tucked away from friction and weather. They also become a canvas for expression. Cowrie shells, beads, threads, and metal cuffs turn a practical style into a story you wear on your head. Lineage, tribe, status, and personal taste can all be signaled in how you part, braid, and decorate.

The products are simple, too. Shea, coconut, palm kernel oil, and sometimes marula or baobab oil are all worked into hair to keep it strong. In East Africa, some people use powdered leaves like qasil mixed with water instead of shampoo. Chebe is mixed with oil and worked into braids in Chad. It's messy and definitely not office-friendly, but it works. Even in harsh climates, many women who use it have long, thick hair. That says something.

There are other rituals, too. In Sudan, some women do *dukhan*, a smoke bath using special woods. You sit on a stool with a cloth around you while the smoke does its thing. People say it makes your skin smoother and leaves a deep scent. Brides and new moms might do it as part of their care. If you didn't grow up with it, it might look intense. But if you did, it's just another way to take care of yourself.

You might see women sitting under a tree, fingers moving steadily as they braid one another's hair. As the sun sets, friends are at the river, taking turns scrubbing each other's backs. Aunties lean over kitchen tables, showing teenagers how to melt shea butter to just the right consistency. They show them how to roll warm sugar. The sugar pulls and stretches between their palms like honey and suddenly feels right in a way you recognize more than understand.

You hear the noise of blow dryers and laughter. Now we are at a city hair salon, where people share stories with their stylists. Looking good and feeling like you belong are both part of the experience. Hair appointments are a time for transformation and a regular chance to see your favorite people.

Modern Takes: Heritage, Business, and Global Influence

These days, African beauty wisdom isn't just hanging on by a thread. It's spreading and turning into real businesses. People are moving from 'imported is better' to 'what we have here is powerful.'

African-owned brands are popping up everywhere. They're whipping shea butter into lighter textures, turning black soap into liquid face wash and shampoo, and mixing local ingredients like moringa and hibiscus with things like niacinamide.

Global brands woke up to what was going on. It's common to see brands touting shea butter from women's cooperatives in Burkina Faso or Ghana. Marketing campaigns talk openly about the women who gather the nuts and the communities that benefit from fair trade. For many buyers, knowing their body cream supports real people as well as their own skin adds another layer of satisfaction.

Social media then made this trend explode, and now, suddenly, everyone wants in.

African net sponges took over social media almost overnight. All you could see were TikTok routines, Reddit threads, and shower restock videos. People posted dramatic before-and-afters, tossed their loofahs, and treated the nets like a brand-new secret. Black soap became the internet's go-to for clearing skin. It was preferred over more expensive products. Sure, there were knockoffs, and some people learned the hard way they still needed moisturizer, but the traditional, grandmother-approved methods were solving what modern products couldn't.

The natural hair movement amplifies African hair care philosophies. What many African women were told to hide or "tame" for years is now being reclaimed as something worthy of care and celebration. Pre-shampoo oil treatments, protective styles, satin bonnets at night, and braids as rest periods for fragile hair. These ideas relate to practices from villages and towns across the continent. They are now discussed in YouTube tutorials, Instagram reels, and books about hair health.

Sun protection is finally getting some attention, too. Older generations thought melanin was enough, but younger people aren't buying it. They want sunscreens that don't leave a gray cast and feel good on their skin, sometimes mixing them with African oils to get it right. Some brands are finally making formulas just for darker skin. The idea being that you deserve sun protection that works for you.

Makeup has followed a similar path.

For years, foundation ranges ignored the full spectrum of darker shades and undertones. Now, local brands in Nigeria, South Africa, Kenya, and beyond are creating products with shades that match the people around them. They know that one deep brown is not enough. They understand that some skins read more golden, others more red, others almost blue. Their palettes, highlighters, and lipsticks are designed to pop on rich skin rather than disappear or look chalky. The result is not just better makeup. It is a better representation.

Using the African Net Sponge: A Daily Ritual for Smoother Skin

If you want to bring a bit of this everyday know-how into your own bathroom, start with the net sponge. It doesn't look like much. But used right, it can change how your skin feels all year.

Here is how to turn it from "just a strip of net" into a small daily ritual.

1. Open and wet the net

Most nets arrive bunched up or tied into a loop. Unfurl it and notice its length. Some stretch longer than your arm span, which is precisely the point. Step into the shower and wet it thoroughly. As water hits it, the net softens but keeps that slight scratchy texture that does the work.

2. Add just a little soap

Squeeze a small amount of body wash onto the net or rub a bar of soap along it a few times. You will quickly see that the net multiplies lather. You do not need much. Work it in with your hands until you have a cushion of foam.

This is one of the quiet gifts of the net. More cleanse, less product.

3. Start scrubbing the easy places

Scrunch the net into a ball and begin with your arms and chest. Use circular or back-and-forth motions, adjusting the pressure so it feels invigorating but not harsh. You will feel the texture immediately. It is not painful, but it does not pretend to be. It gets right to the point.

Move to your legs, feet, and hands. On rougher spots like elbows, knees, and heels, you can press a little more firmly. Think of it as polishing, not attacking.

4. Stretch it for your back

This is where the length shines. Hold one end of the net in each hand and stretch it across your back like a towel. Gently see-saw it up and down. No twisting, no asking someone else to help. Upper back, mid back, lower back, all get their turn.

5. Rinse, notice, and moisturize

Rinse your body thoroughly. As the soap and loosened skin wash away, feel your arms and legs with your hands. They'll often feel cleaner than they have in a long time, that "squeaky" kind of clean that's only satisfying if you follow it with moisture.

Step out, pat yourself dry, and apply a body cream or oil while your skin is still slightly damp. This is where shea butter, coconut oil, or your favorite lotion comes in. After a week or two of this routine, you might notice your usual moisturizer suddenly seems to work better. Really, it's just reaching skin that isn't covered in a layer of old cells anymore.

6. Rinse and hang the net

Hold the net under the shower and squeeze it a few times to rinse off the soap. Then hang it where air can reach it on all sides. Within a short time, it will be completely dry. That quick-drying is why it stays fresh with little effort. No damp, sour smell. No hidden mildew.

A single net can last months, even a year, before the texture softens too much and you decide to replace it.

7. Find your own rhythm

A lot of people in West and Central Africa use the net sponge every day with no trouble. If your skin is sensitive, start with two or three times a week and see how it feels. There's no medal for the most aggressive scrubbing. The goal is consistent, gentle exfoliation that keeps your skin smooth over time.

Once you get used to it, you might notice something subtle.

Your shower stops feeling like just another chore squeezed between tasks and starts to feel like a little reset button you press for yourself. You move the net over your skin, watch the lather foam and fade, feel the warmth of the water and the buzz of circulation under your skin. Then you step out, moisturize, get dressed, and carry that quiet sense of 'I took care of myself today' into the rest of your life.

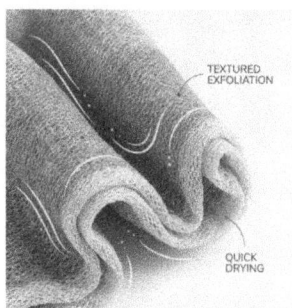

In real life, modern routines are a mix. A woman in Kampala might wash her face with black soap, follow with a Korean-style essence, slap on a French moisturizer, then seal everything with raw shea at night. A man in Accra might get his beard lined at a trendy barbershop, then go home and rub in a simple shea and coconut oil blend his grandmother swears by.

That's what these African rituals have always done at their core. They take ordinary ingredients, simple tools, and everyday moments and turn them into quiet declarations of worth. And that, more than any product label or marketing campaign, is the kind of beauty that lasts.

There's a quiet confidence in that.

CHAPTER 6

Latin America – Herbal Baths, Kitchen Cures, and Rhythms of Beauty

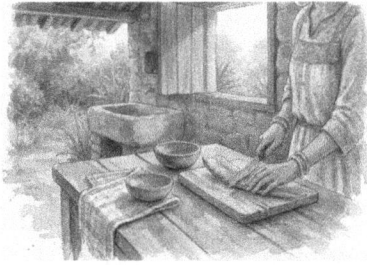

In Mexico, a grandmother is working aloe through her granddaughter's hair. She's promising it'll shine all day. In Peru, the steam is doing its thing as someone is soaking in a hot bath with muña leaves. A guy on the beach in the Caribbean scrubs his arms with coffee and brown sugar and then rinses off in the ocean. They're everyday routines that work.

Across Latin America, beauty routines blend Indigenous wisdom, Spanish, and African traditions. These habits are all about looking good, feeling comfortable, and staying protected. They are about seeking a little joy in the everyday. So let's begin.

Traditional Practices: From Rainforest Wisdom to Kitchen Remedies

Latin America covers a vast area, from Mexico all the way down to Patagonia and out to the Caribbean. The beauty routines are just as varied. Most of these traditions start at home, passed down by family, and they usually begin with plants. These are the herbs, fruits, and roots that people use instead of store-bought lotions or serums.

Herbal Baths & Cleansing Rituals

Take Mexico's *temazcal*, for example. It's a dome-shaped steam lodge where people sweat it out with herbs and hot stones, letting go of stress and starting fresh. Even if you're not in a steam lodge, you'll find families pouring chamomile over kids' hair for shine, tossing rosemary and rue into bathwater for a boost, or boiling eucalyptus leaves for a quick decongesting steam at home.

Long before modern products hit the shelves, Indigenous groups across Central and South America just used what was around them. Amazonian women washed with clay instead of soap or shampoo. Buriti palm oil, bright orange and loaded with nutrients, was their go-to for protecting skin and hair from the sun. Still is.

Glow, Smoothness, and Everyday Radiance

If there's one thing Latin beauty is known for, it's that healthy glow. Grandmothers knew how to exfoliate and brighten skin way before spas made it trendy:

Coffee grounds mixed with coconut oil for firming, brightening, and waking up the skin.

Brown sugar and lemon to soften elbows and knees.

Fruit-based treatments are everywhere. Papaya gets mashed up for face masks because its enzymes smooth your skin. Cacao, which the Aztecs and Mayans considered sacred, is used as a moisturizer or scrub. And avocado is basically its own beauty category. People use it to hydrate both skin and hair.

Hair Traditions: Nourish, Shine, and Social Ritual

Hair care is a big deal in Latin America. In the Dominican Republic, going to the salon every week is almost mandatory and it's a social event. Hair gets deep conditioned, rolled, dried, and styled with the kind of skill that's been passed down for generations.

At home, families rely on what's in the kitchen:

Aloe vera to detangle and soothe the scalp.

Avocado masks to restore moisture.

Mayonnaise or olive oil for deep conditioning.

Beer rinses for shine and body.

Indigenous and Afro-Latin communities have their own go-to routines. Items like coconut milk masks and clay cleansers are staples. These are the kinds of things mixed quietly at home. Now, everyone's catching on.

Scent, Ritual, and Colonial Echoes

Caribbean grooming has its own unmistakable signature: bay rum. Steeped in alcohol with spices and bay leaves, it became the region's classic post-shave splash — bright, spicy, and unmistakably "clean." It's still used in barbershops today, alongside modern tools and global trends.

Folklore also blends with grooming. Floral baths with marigold or rosemary may be prescribed by a healer to release negative energy. As a bonus, they promise to leave the skin glowing. Beauty and spiritual health walk side by side, one improving the other.

Modern Fusion: New Trends, Old Roots

Now, the beauty world is looking back to Latin America. The same things grandmothers used in their kitchens are popping up in fancy bottles everywhere. *Açaí* from Brazil, *maracuyá* oil from the Amazon, *quinoa* from the Andes. They're all in high-end products now.

But inside Latin America, the movement is just as strong. Young people are taking old ingredients and building new brands around them. Brazilian companies are all about Amazonian oils. Peruvian coca-leaf scrubs are offered right next to Swedish massage.

The Influence of Social Media

Beauty influencers across Latin America are mixing tradition with viral trends:

A creator pairs a Korean snail cream with her Colombian grandmother's rice water toner.

Dominican natural hair influencers teach curl care using passionfruit masks and coconut-water spritzes.

These are little ways people hope to keep heritage alive, with a new twist.

Men's Grooming: Blending Old & New

In barbershops from Puerto Rico to São Paulo, people are making their own form of art. Modern fades and beard shaping are followed by classic touches like hot towels and splashes of bay rum. Many barbers blend local remedies like aloe, rosemary oil, coconut oil into their services. Grooming is cultural, stylish, and proudly Latin.

Shifting Beauty Ideals

Latin America's beauty standards are changing. Afro-Latin and Indigenous beauty are finally being celebrated, and natural hair movements have reshaped entire industries. In places once ruled by relaxers and straightening treatments, curls and coils now shine in all their patterns.

Younger generations are claiming what was always theirs. A diverse, multicultural look built on certainty, creativity, and roots.

DIY Ritual: Abuela's Avocado Hair Mask

If you want to try a classic Latin beauty ritual, make this deeply nourishing mask. It is a favorite in kitchens across the region.

You'll Need:

1 ripe avocado
2 tbsp olive or coconut oil
1 egg yolk
Optional: 1 tbsp honey; a few drops of rosemary oil

How to Mix:

Mash the avocado until creamy. Add oil, egg yolk, and honey (if using) and mix until smooth.

Instructions:

Apply to dry or slightly damp hair and comb through for even coverage.

Cover your hair with a shower cap and let it sit for 20 to 30 minutes.

Rinse hair thoroughly with lukewarm water.

Shampoo your hair well and condition lightly.

Why It Works:

Avocado hydrates, oil nourishes, egg strengthens, and honey pulls in moisture. The result is softer, shinier, and happier hair.

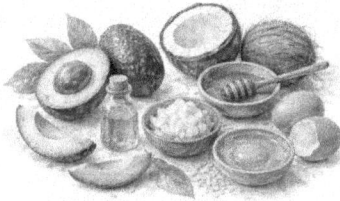

The Heart of Latin Beauty

Latin beauty rituals are lively, fragrant, and full of personality. They're done to salsa music, in crowded kitchens, in steamy bathhouses, on breezy porches, and beside rivers. They exist to soothe and to celebrate. They remind us that beauty does not have to be quiet or clinical. Sometimes it is vibrant, communal, sensual, and wonderfully simple.

And always, always, crafted with love.

CHAPTER 7

Europe – Old World Elegance and Country Comforts

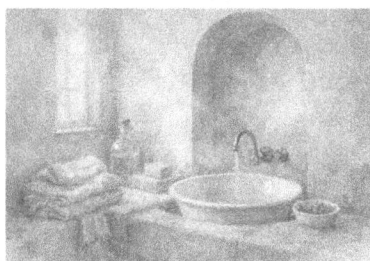

Picture this: Romans lounging in warm, oil-scented baths, their voices bouncing off marble ceilings. In Provence, someone's grandmother is picking lavender and rosemary to toss in her washbasin, just like her mother and grandmother did. European beauty rituals can be over-the-top or dead simple, but they all have one thing in common: for ages people have mixed science, art, and whatever they could find in nature to take care of themselves.

Traditional Practices: From the Mediterranean to the North Sea

Europe is a patchwork of cultures, each with its own beauty secrets. But some things show up repeatedly. Communal baths? Thank the Romans for that. The word 'spa' even comes from a Belgian town famous for its baths since Roman times. And then there's the love of herbs and simple, homemade remedies. Chamomile in the east, olive oil in the south. No matter where you go, you'll find people using what's around them to look and feel their best.

Let's start in the south, where olive oil is basically a way of life. The ancient Greeks and Romans used it for everything. They cleansed their skin, used it for moisturizing, even mixed it with herbs for extra benefits.

Castile soap from Spain? That's just olive oil soap, and it's been around since at least the 1500s. People in Greece, Italy, and Spain have washed with it for generations. Now, it's a product in stores, but it started as a simple staple. Want shiny hair? Warm up some olive oil, comb it through, wrap your head in a towel, wait an hour, and wash it out. Your hair will feel amazing. Italian grandmas still rub a little olive oil into their cuticles and elbows at night. Ask a Mediterranean grandmother her secret to smooth skin, and she'll probably say olive oil, and maybe a glass of red wine, but that's another story.

And yes, wine isn't just for drinking. In France, people used to bathe in the leftover grape mush after winemaking, thinking it would boost their health, or maybe they just liked the smell. Grapes are packed with antioxidants, so they were onto something. In Germany and Czechia, people soaked in warm beer for softer skin and less stress. The yeast is good for your skin, too. These days, you can go to a beer spa in Prague, sit in a tub of beer, and even sip a pint while you soak. Only in Europe, right?

Head north and you'll find the sauna (or Russian *banya*) at the center of self-care. In Finland, people sweat in dry heat, then roll in the snow or jump into icy water. That hot-cold shock? It's supposed to boost your circulation and immunity.

They even beat themselves, or each other, with bundles of birch or oak leaves. Sounds intense, but it scrubs your skin, and the oils help sore muscles. Afterward, you rinse off and feel like a new person. Many Finns swear their clear skin and strong health come from weekly sauna sessions. They call the sauna the poor man's pharmacy. Spas everywhere now offer 'Nordic spa' routines, but in Finland, it's just what Europe's spa towns have been around forever. Places like Baden-Baden, Vichy, Karlovy Vary, and Bath all grew up around natural springs and muds that people thought could cure just about anything or at least make you look better.

Back in the 1800s, the rich and fancy would travel for weeks just to 'take the waters.' Translation: drink weird mineral tonics, soak in hot baths, and get slathered in mud. It wasn't just about health—it was a social scene and a beauty ritual rolled into one. And guess what? A lot of those traditions are still alive. People still line up at Budapest's baths or Italy's terme to soak in sulfur-rich water for their skin or sore muscles.

The modern beauty industry jumped on this, too. France's Vichy brand began with Vichy's mineral springs. La Roche-Posay began with spring water from their village. Now, they bottle that water in sprays and base their creams on it, promising soothing, anti-redness benefits— basically, a mini spa at home. For decades, European women have sworn by spritzing thermal spring water on their faces after cleansing to calm the skin. Even if it seems like just fancy water, the minerals do have a soothing effect.

Herbal knowledge across Europe is too vast to cover fully, but some highlights:

In Central and Eastern Europe, chamomile (or manzanilla) is the go-to herb for just about everything. People use it in baths to calm their skin, as a rinse to brighten blonde hair, and even as a compress for puffy eyes.

Rosemary was a big deal in Mediterranean Europe. There's even a legendary recipe called Queen of Hungary's Water—a medieval tonic made with rosemary and herbs, believed to be a youth elixir and maybe the first real cosmetic toner. These days, rosemary is known for its antimicrobial and stimulating powers, and you'll spot it in scalp tonics and toners. And yes, 'Hungarian water' still pops up in fancy perfumes.

Lavender has been used in France and England since at least the Middle Ages for scenting bathwater, washing linens, and in skincare (its antiseptic properties made it a staple in facial steams for acne or minor cuts).

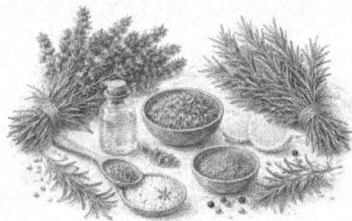

In Scandinavia, aside from sauna, you had folk remedies like brewer's yeast masks (from the beer brewing tradition, to clear complexion) and sour milk baths (the lactic acid would gently exfoliate. Rumor has it Cleopatra did it, but country milkmaids also knew milk made their hands soft).

Seaweed wraps were coastal Europe's secret. Ireland and Brittany (France) have used seaweed in baths for skin detox and softness for ages; today, "thalassotherapy" (sea therapy) resorts in France incorporate algae masks and saltwater pools exactly in that tradition.

Men in Europe had their grooming traditions too:

Barbering was an art. The classic Western barbershop experience includes a hot towel, straight razor shave, maybe a splash of cologne. It is a tradition that thrived in Europe. Eau de Cologne, is a light citrus-and-herb scent that men and women used liberally to freshen up. They'd even mix it with water for a quick cleaning wipe-down or gargle it as mouthwash.

In Victorian England, there were moustache waxes and hair pomades aplenty; these often-contained natural waxes like beeswax or macassar oil (from the Makassar island palm oil). Interestingly, that "macassar oil" was so commonly used that antimacassars (chair cloths) were invented to protect furniture from men's hair oil stains!

Dry brushing the skin with a natural-bristle brush (to exfoliate and improve circulation) is a European practice that many credit to the ancient Greeks or, later, to Scandinavians, but it became a spa staple in Europe by the mid-20th century. Now, lots of people worldwide do dry body brushing as part of a wellness routine (especially before showering, to supposedly help lymph flow – something Finnish grandmothers did with a rough washcloth in sauna generations ago).

These days, Europe's beauty industry is high-tech. Think French skincare labs and Italian hair products. But people are also rediscovering old-school remedies. 'Apothecary skincare' and 'heritage brands' are suddenly cool again. Kiehl's started as a European-style pharmacy in New York, and Santa Maria Novella in Italy has been making rosewater and violet creams since the 1600s. Walk into any European drugstore, and you'll still find pure rosewater and castor oil on the shelves. Rosewater is a classic toner or linen spray, and castor oil has always been used to strengthen hair and lashes. Now it's even in brow serums and mascaras.

People love to mix old and new in their routines. Picture this: a Parisian starts her day with vitamin C serum, but at night she washes her face with plain olive oil soap, just like her grandmother did. A Swedish teenager still takes a weekly bath with pine tar soap because his grandfather swore it kept his skin clear. He might even try out a trendy 10-step skincare routine on top of that. Some habits just stick around, no matter what's trending.

One thing you notice in Europe is the focus on moderation and consistency. Sure, some people have elaborate daily rituals, but most stick to the basics: cleanse, moisturize, protect. Maybe a face mask on Sunday night, or a facial at the salon once a month. This whole 'less but better' mindset is catching on everywhere. The new 'skinimalism' trend, that is using fewer products so your skin can breathe, fits right in with the classic French or

Scandinavian approach: a few good products and a healthy lifestyle.

Of course, not everyone in Europe does things the same way. A stylish woman in Madrid might have a dozen products lined up on her vanity. Someone in rural Poland might just use cold cream and chamomile water. That's the beauty of it. You get both: luxury creams from Switzerland and simple, time-tested tricks like a Greek yogurt and honey face mask for clear skin.

Maybe that's the real secret in Europe: balance. Science and nature, luxury and practicality, old traditions and new ideas and all of it working together.

DIY Rosewater Toner: Timeless European Elixir

Rosewater is one of Europe's oldest and simplest beauty tricks. It's a gentle toner and smells amazing. Want to try it yourself? You can make a basic version at home and get a little old-world elegance in your routine.

What you'll need: about 2 cups of fresh, fragrant rose petals (make sure they're not sprayed with pesticides) and 2.5 cups of distilled water. No fresh roses? Use about 1 cup of dried rose buds, the kind sold for tea works great.

Method 1: Infusion. Think of it like making strong rose tea. Put the petals in a heatproof bowl or pot. Boil the distilled water and pour it over the petals. Just enough to cover them. Cover with a lid or plate to keep the steam (and the scent) in. Let it cool to room temperature. The water will turn pale pink or gold and smell amazing. Strain out the petals, pour the rosewater into a clean glass bottle, and keep it in the fridge. It'll last about a week. This simple toner has long been a European favorite. The toner is gentle, soothing, and just a little bit extra.

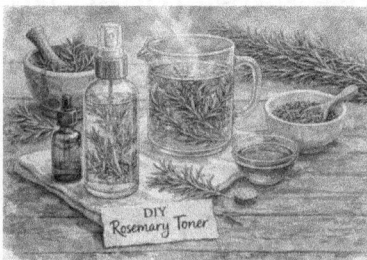

DIY Rosemary Toner

Method 2: Distillation (the stovetop hack). Want rosewater that lasts longer? Try this. Put a heavy ramekin or brick in the middle of a big pot. Scatter the rose petals around it and add distilled water until the petals are just covered (don't cover the top of the brick). Set a metal bowl on the brick to catch the drips. Put the lid on the pot upside down. Bring the water to a simmer. Pile some ice cubes on top of the lid. The cold helps the steam turn back into water and drip into the bowl. You'll hear it dripping. Keep going for 20-30 minutes, adding more ice if needed. When you're done, carefully take out the bowl. That's your pure, distilled rosewater. It'll keep for a few months in the fridge.

How to use it: Store your rosewater in a glass bottle. Amber or blue colored bottles are best to keep out the light. To use as a toner, pour some on a cotton pad and swipe it over your face after cleansing. It'll pick up any leftover dirt, tighten your pores a bit, and leave your skin soft and smelling like a rose garden. No need to rinse—just let it dry. You can also pour it into a spray bottle and mist your face whenever you need a pick-me-up. The scent is a mood booster. For tired eyes, soak cotton pads in chilled rosewater and lay them over your eyes. It's an old European trick for puffy eyes after a rough night.

Want to level up? Add a few drops of glycerin to your rosewater for extra moisture. That's a trick from Victorian times. Or mix in some witch hazel for even more pore-tightening power, while still keeping that incredible scent.

When you make and use rosewater, you're joining a tradition that goes back centuries. Everyone from queens to country folk has loved it. It's simple, but it feels special. Picture Marie Antoinette dabbing it on her face, or a medieval herbalist making it for a queen. Every time you catch that rose scent, you're connected with history. Imagine Persian gardens, Italian monasteries, and English cottages. In one splash, you get a little piece of Europe's beauty story.

This DIY is easy to follow and honestly, who wouldn't want to feel like they're in a Jane Austen novel, dabbing rosewater on their wrists? The best skincare is often natural and straightforward. Europeans have always used what grows around them to look and feel good. The fact that rosewater is still a favorite—now in fancy sprays and creams—shows some traditions never go out of style. Enjoy the soft skin and subtle scent and treat yourself to a bit of old-world luxury that barely costs a thing.

CHAPTER 8

United States – Melting Pot of Modern Routines

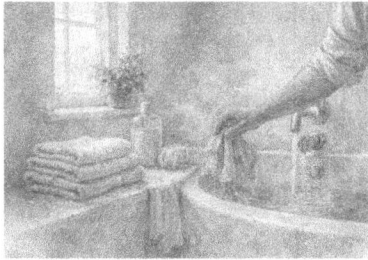

Imagine this: someone in Manhattan is ending their day with a cleanser from Seoul, a toner from Paris, and a turmeric mask they found on TikTok. Meanwhile, in Alabama, an older man is washing up with a bar of lye soap he made himself from fat and ash, just like his mom did when money was tight, but there was always soap.

Two lives. Two counters. One country.

That's America for you. Beauty here isn't some neat tradition passed down without a scratch. It's a mix of what people brought, what they found, what they made up, and what they clung to when things got tough. Old tricks live right next to new serums. Native plant know-how is still around, even if marketing tries to shout over it. And let's be honest: under almost every routine is the same question. What if something else works better?

There's no single American beauty tradition. There are dozens, all stacked on top of each other.

Indigenous nations had their own ways of caring for skin and hair long before anyone called this place America. Then people came from everywhere—Europe, Africa, Asia, Latin America. Each group brought their routines, shaped them to fit this land, and handed them down in kitchens, backyards, and crowded apartments.

If you want to start somewhere, look at Native communities. In the Southwest, tribes washed their hair with yucca root, making a gentle lather right from the plant. Others mixed animal fats and local herbs for salves and hair dressings, or used cornmeal as both food and a way to scrub skin smooth. Sweat lodges filled with cedar and sage steam weren't about pampering. They were how you cleaned body and spirit with what you had, in the place you lived.

Enslaved Africans brought their own knowledge but had to adapt it to new ground. Oils, braids, protective styles, scalp care rituals all crossed the ocean and changed to fit whatever plants and products were around. Later, when freedom was mostly a promise, Black entrepreneurs built an entire industry on that wisdom.

Women like Madam C. J. Walker and Annie Malone offered more than tins of pomade. They created systems involving regular washing, scalp massage, and deliberate styling. All of this was very important because this came at a time when Black women were often denied access to basic grooming spaces. Their formulas combined new industrial ingredients, such as petrolatum, with familiar ones, such as castor and coconut oil. The real innovation, though, was that your hair deserves consistent, intentional care.

European settlers brought their own habits, then had to sort things out. On farms, soap was a rough block of animal fat and ashes that cleaned everything from clothes to floors, kids to dishes. No luxury, no fancy scent, just pure function. People noticed it calmed poison ivy and bug bites, so it doubled as medicine. Vinegar rinses cut through soap scum and make hair shinier. Baking soda was another miracle product because it did everything. People used it to brush teeth, scrub sinks, and freshen underarms. This was beauty by necessity. Use what you have and make it last.

Not every story is rugged and muddy, though. Religious communities like the Shakers grew meticulous herb gardens and sold rosewater, lavender water, and salves. This was early American "clean beauty" before the phrase existed. As cities expanded, companies like Pond's and Avon bottled creams and tonics that promised refinement beyond home remedies. The shelves changed, but the home tricks never really left.

When money ran out, people got creative. During the Great Depression, stockings were a luxury. So, women darkened their legs with tea or kitchen drippings and drew a fake seam up the back with a pencil. Cold creams like Noxzema did it all. It took off makeup, soothed sunburns, worked as night cream. One jar did the job of half your bathroom shelf today.

Over decades, a toolbox of distinctly American staples settled in:

Oatmeal baths to calm rashes and chickenpox itch.

Witch hazel for bug bites, oily T-zones, and mysterious bruises.

Epsom salts to soak sore muscles and soften rough heels.

Petroleum jelly for lips, knuckles, cuticles, minor burns, cracked nostrils in winter, and even as an emergency shoe polish.

Milk of magnesia, technically a laxative, repurposed as a mattifying mask in pageant circles and backstage dressing rooms.

New waves of immigrants quietly stretched that kit even further. Eastern Europeans brought steam baths that became city bathhouses and, later, spa culture. Chinese communities shared herbal tonics and roots that, decades later, ended up in supplements and skincare. Mexican and Central American families used aloe vera for burns and scalp care long before it turned into neon-green gel on every drugstore shelf.

In recent decades, Asian innovation arrived in a louder, shinier way. South Korean and Japanese brands made double cleansing, hydrating toners, sheet masks for Friday nights, and sunscreens that feel like skincare, not chalk, part of the routine. Latin American traditions turned avocado masks, sugar scrubs, and coffee grounds into obvious self-care, not odd experiments.

Men's grooming followed its own crooked path.

It started with classic barbershops: striped poles, hot lather, straight razors, aftershaves that smelled like spice and hope. Then came sideburns and mustaches in the '60s and '70s. The 2000s brought cologne-and-gel minimalism. Now? It's a remix. Barbers shape beards with sharp precision under LED ring lights, then wrap a hot towel around your face like it's 1925. Old rituals returned, just with better playlists and cleaner fades.

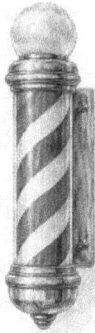

Even spa culture is a patchwork. A massage menu might mix Swedish moves with Himalayan salt stones, then add a Reiki session in a dim room. Korean spas in Los Angeles scrub years of dead skin off people whose grandparents never left the Midwest. Sweat lodges, infrared saunas, float tanks are pieces borrowed from everywhere, all on one map.

Somewhere along the way, self-care became the American way to frame it. The phrase is new, but the instinct isn't. Routines stopped being just about looking good for other people and started being about staying sane and okay for yourself. Put your phone down. Run a bath. Put on a mask. Light a candle and call it medicine for your nerves. That shift changed how a lot of us look in the mirror.

Trying to name one American routine is like trying to name one American meal. It depends on who you ask, where they grew up, what they can afford, and what their algorithm keeps tossing at them. But some patterns keep popping up.

First: the mix-and-match counter.

A cleanser from Tokyo and an acid toner from a French pharmacy. A retinol serum from a New Jersey lab. A moisturizer with shea butter sourced from a Ghanaian women's co-op. A sunscreen using Korean filter tech. The shelf looks like a tiny United Nations. Brand loyalty is optional; curation is everything. People assemble their own systems one bottle at a time.

Second: the chase for results.

Americans are excellent at turning self-improvement into a project. The internet is flooded with "glow-up" videos and routines stretched. Double cleansing at night. Weekly exfoliants. At-home devices that buzz, pulse, or flash a red light. Sometimes, it's too much and skin rebels with all the over-exfoliation, barrier damage, and peeling noses. That overdoing becomes its own lesson, pushing some people toward gentler, fewer-step routines. The pendulum swings between maximalist and minimalist, and most of us live somewhere in the middle.

Third: a serious push toward inclusivity.

For a long time, beauty ads and shade ranges ignored huge swaths of the population. Foundations stopped about three shades into "tan." Hair products were available in one or two textures. When brands finally launched broad foundation lines with dozens of shades and haircare grouped by curl pattern and coil type, it didn't just change shelves—it shifted stories.

Black, Latino, Asian, Indigenous, and mixed-race communities pushed hard to be centered instead of tacked on. That insistence reshaped everyday routines: multi-step curl-care wash days, protective styles layered with creams and oils, sunscreens that don't leave a gray film on deeper skin, product labels that say "4C coils" instead of "all hair types." Bathroom counters now quietly document those battles and wins.

Fourth: men's routines are expanding.

Younger men are far more likely to cleanse, moisturize, treat acne marks, and apply SPF without apology. Beard oils soften both hair and ego. It's normal to see a guy in a sheet mask on the couch or getting a brow cleanup and mini-facial at the barbershop. Grooming becomes less about hiding the fact that you care and more about feeling comfortable in your skin.

Fifth: the DIY streak, upgraded.

That pioneer "figure it out yourself" energy never left; it just picked up Pinterest boards, YouTube, and ring lights. People mix sugar scrubs in mason jars, pour bath bombs into silicone molds, stir coffee grounds into coconut oil, and rebrand it as "Sunday spa." Some recipes come from grandmas. Others come from strangers on the internet. A few get retired after a sticky disaster. The survivors become mini rituals: the lip scrub every December, the oatmeal soak for itchy kids, the vinegar rinse after a month of heavy products.

Sixth: tech in the bathroom.

Of course, gadgets made their way into skincare. Apps track how long you've been on retinol. Smart mirrors say they can analyze your pores. Devices promise to tone, lift, zap, or smooth. For some people, it's too much. For others, it's a little comforting. If you can press a button and see data, maybe you're finally doing this whole "taking care of yourself" thing right.

People talk openly about how their skin changed when they slept more, drank less, took meds, went to therapy, or changed their diet. Collagen in coffee, greens powders in smoothies, yoga for stress, SPF every morning, thick balm at night. The moisturizer becomes one tile in a bigger mosaic: mental health, movement, food, rest, and products all in conversation.

But there's something quieter going on. It's not about being perfect. It's about giving yourself permission.

Permission to try things. Permission to borrow ideas from other cultures and give credit.

Permission to toss what doesn't work, keep what does, and claim a little time for yourself. Even on the days when you don't love what you see in the mirror.

One of the subtler pleasures in this whole messy, generous beauty landscape is building a smell that feels like you. Americans borrowed the idea of layering fragrance from places where it's been an art, and then did what they always do: tinkered with it until it felt personal.

Here's a simple way to experiment with scent layering without turning your bathroom into a fog of perfume.

1. **Start with a base.**

Right after you shower, while your skin is still slightly damp, apply body lotion or oil. Choose something with a soft, simple scent or with notes that match your main perfume: vanilla, coconut, almond, clean musk, a sheer floral, or even unscented if you're cautious.

This base does two jobs at once: It moisturizes, so scent clings longer. It sets a quiet background note for everything else to rest on. Think of it as painting the wall a neutral tone before hanging art.

2. Add your main perfume.

Next, apply your primary fragrance to pulse points: wrists, inner elbows, neck, behind the ears, maybe the back of the knees if you want a subtle trail.

Spray or dab, then resist the urge to rub your wrists together. Friction can heat the skin and make the top notes burn off faster. Let the perfume blossom on its own as you move.

The base and the perfume are already interacting. Vanilla lotion can warm up a sharp floral. A clean musk body cream can make a citrus scent feel more like skin and less like a cleaning spray.

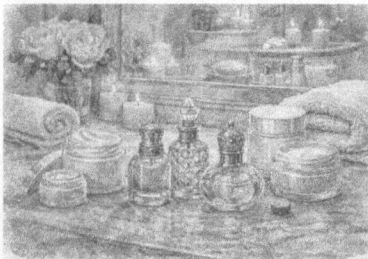

3. Optional top note.

If you feel playful, add one more layer: a light body mist or a sheer cologne. This light fragrance layer should be more transparent than your main perfume, something bright, airy, or green. Mist it lightly over your hair or clothes, or spray once into the air and walk through. You'll notice it mainly in the first hour. After that, it fades, leaving the base and main scent to do the heavy lifting. It's like squeezing lemon over a dish just before serving it. The food was already seasoned; you're just adding lift.

4. Adjust as the day unfolds.

Fragrance shifts over time. Morning brings sparkly top notes. Afternoon moves into the softer woods, musks, or vanillas. Heat makes scent bloom; cold keeps it close.

If you want a midday refresh, reach for a travel spray of your main perfume or a tiny roll-on oil that echoes one of its notes (rose, vanilla, citrus, sandalwood). Tap a little onto pulse points. You're not rebuilding the whole structure, just nudging it awake.

Notice how the environment affects it: office air-conditioning can flatten a delicate scent; a crowded subway can make it feel louder than you planned. Paying attention like this quietly turns "putting on perfume" into a small mindfulness exercise.

5.   Let it become yours.

The fundamental goal of layering isn't to smell strong. It's to smell like yourself on purpose.

6. Over time, you'll find combinations you keep reaching for:

Creamy vanilla lotion under orange blossom perfume.

Sandalwood oil has a rose fragrance.

Clean cotton base under something musky and warm.

Someone might say, "You always smell amazing—what is that?" and you'll end up telling a small story instead of naming a single bottle: "It's this lotion, plus that perfume, and sometimes a little citrus spray." That story is the whole point.

You gathered influences from everywhere and arranged them into something that reads, unmistakably, as you.

In a country where routines are always changing, shelves are packed, and advice never stops, taking a few minutes to layer your scent on purpose is its own kind of calm. It's a small daily ritual.

You get to make this up as you go. You can change your mind. You're allowed to enjoy it.

CHAPTER 9

Perfume – Scent Rituals

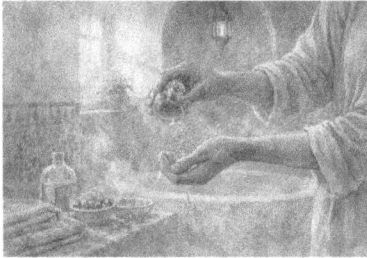

In the Bronx, New York, a young woman unboxes a fragrance that went viral on TikTok. She sprays the air and walks through the mist. She grins as pear, vanilla, and clean musks settle on her skin. Thousands of miles away, in a small workshop in rural Oman, an older man starts his morning distilling rose petals, repeating the same steps his father and grandfather taught him.

They'll never meet, but they're both doing something simple and powerful: turning the air around them into a feeling you can sense.

Fragrance is the quiet thread running through everything in this book. We've talked about baths, oils, scrubs, masks, and hair rituals. Scent has been there the whole time mixed into black soap, floating in steam, hidden in butters and herbs. This chapter pulls it forward. We'll look at how perfume began, how it works, why certain scents feel the way they do, what's happening with viral trends, Arabian fragrance houses, dupe brands, collecting perfume as a hobby, and how to choose scents that honestly feel like you.

Don't worry, this isn't a chemistry test. Think of it as a quick tour through the world of perfume, just enough to help you find your way without getting overwhelmed.

Humans + Smell: A Very Short History

Long before anyone argued about "beast mode projection" on YouTube, humans were already perfuming themselves.

The word "perfume" comes from Latin for "through smoke." Early fragrance was not a bottle on a dresser; it was incense rising from charcoal and disappearing into the sky. People burned resins and woods as offerings to gods, as air fresheners in crowded cities, and as a way to feel closer to something sacred.

In ancient Mesopotamia, a woman named Tapputi, one of the first recorded chemists, was distilling flowers, oils, and resins into scented balms.

In Egypt, people anointed their bodies with perfumed oils for worship, beauty, and, honestly, to survive the heat.

Greeks and Romans slathered themselves in aromatic oils and powders. For them, scent was about status and pleasure.

During the Islamic Golden Age, making perfume became both a craft and a careful process. Experts improved ways to extract scents, wrote down recipes, and tried out roses, oud, and many herbs.

Then the knowledge moved again through trade, conquest, and curiosity into Europe, where Italian and French courts turned perfume into a luxury symbol and eventually a full-blown industry.

There's a pattern: every culture took what came before, added their own favorite plants and ideas, and passed it along. We're just the latest ones to pick up the thread.

How Perfume Works: Notes and Layers

Have you ever sprayed something you loved in the store, only to hate it two hours later? Then it turns out you've met the fragrance pyramid.

Perfume isn't one flat smell. It's built in layers called notes:

Top notes – the first hit you smell. Light and loud: citrus, herbs, some fruits, airy florals. They grab your attention and evaporate fast.

Heart (middle) notes – show up once the top settles. These notes are the "personality" of the scent: florals, spices, fruits, tea notes, and some woods.

Base notes – are what's left hours later. Deep and heavy: woods, resins, musks, ambers, vanilla, leather. They're the foundation.

Imagine it like a song:

The top notes are the catchy intro.

The heart is the chorus you keep humming.

The base is the bassline that never really stops.

Why this matters:

Timing. Something bright and lemony at 9 a.m. might be a warm, musky whisper by noon. One fragrance can feel like three different moods depending on when you sniff it.

Skin chemistry. Your skin is not a paper strip. Oils, hormones, diet, even medication, can nudge notes in different directions. That's why the same perfume smells softly sexy on your friend and oddly sour on you.

Once you know perfume has layers, you stop judging in the first two seconds. You let the scent tell its whole story before you decide.

Strength Levels: Why Some Scents Shout and Others Whisper

Another basic that changes everything: concentration.

All perfume is essentially scent + solvent (usually alcohol). The amount of aromatic oil in that mix affects how strong and long-lasting it is:

Extrait / Pure Parfum

Very high concentration. Rich, dense, a few dabs go a long way. Often sits close to the skin but lasts for hours and hours.

Eau de Parfum (EDP)

Medium-high strength. One of the most common formats. Noticeable, lasts several hours, good for day or night.

Eau de Toilette (EDT)

Lighter. Great for daytime, hot weather, or people who prefer a subtle trail.

Eau de Cologne / Body Mist / Splash

Very light, often fresh and citrusy. You'll probably reapply every few hours.

A higher concentration doesn't always mean better. It just means more. If you work close to others or get headaches from strong scents, a light EDT might be your best friend. If you want a scent that lingers on your scarf for days, parfum makes more sense.

The trick is to match the strength of your perfume to your real life, not to what someone else thinks is fancy.

Fragrance Families: How Smells Get Personalities

Perfumers group scents into broad families, so we're not wandering the store completely blindfolded. You'll see different diagrams, but they mostly circle the same big categories:

Simple Beginner Accords

Citrus Blend	Floral Blend	Woody Blend	Gourmand Blend
Bright, zesty, uplifting and fresh.	Romantic, delicate, soft and feminine.	Warm, earthy, rich and comforting.	Sweet, edible, delicious and cozy.

Fresh / Citrus / Green

Lemon, bergamot, lime, herbs, cut grass, and tomato leaf.
Feels like: clean, sharp, energized, air-conditioned. Morning showers, hot days, "I don't want anything heavy."

Floral
Rose, jasmine, tuberose, orange blossom, lily, peony, violet.
Feels like: romantic, polished, soft, sometimes vast and dramatic. Anywhere from "fresh bouquet" to "flower shop explosion."

Woody

Cedar, sandalwood, vetiver, patchouli, pine.
Feels like: grounded, calm, contemplative, sometimes smoky or spicy. Great for cozy moods and cooler weather.

Amber / Oriental

Vanilla, resins, spices, incense, and amber accords

Feels like: warm, plush, sensual, enveloping. It's the fragrance version of a low-lit room and deep cushions.

Gourmand

Vanilla, caramel, chocolate, coffee, almond, sugar, and maple. Feels like: edible. Cozy, playful, sometimes decadent. It can be "bakery" or "grown-up dessert," depending on how it's blended.

Most modern perfumes mix things up: a citrusy top, a floral heart, an amber base. But once you know what you like, shopping for scent gets a lot less overwhelming.

You might learn:

"I love citrus, but only if there's something warm layered under it."

"White florals make me feel over-perfumed; I prefer roses and peonies."

"Woody scents make me feel like myself."

That's the good part. That's you listening to what your own nose likes.

What's Trending: Notes and Vibes Right Now

Fragrance trends move like fashion. A few currents swirling around lately:

Soft gourmands. Vanilla is having a big second life, but less "cupcake," more "vanilla + woods + musk." Think cozy, skin-like sweetness instead of pure sugar.

Green and herbal. Basil, mint, tea leaves, tomato vine, fig leaf. People want scents that feel like fresh air, gardens, and "touch grass" energy.

Airy woods and ambers. Clean sandalwood, modern amber, cashmere woods—warm but not heavy, unisex, office-safe, easy to love.

Skin scents. Musks, ambrette, iris, "your skin but better" blends. These smell like a warm sweater and clean skin, not an obvious "perfume cloud."

Aquatic and salty. Sea sprays, mineral notes, "rain on pavement," "wet stone." Basically, bottled cleanliness plus a little drama.

There's also a big push toward refillable bottles, lighter packaging, and transparency about what's actually in the juice. People want to smell good and feel okay about how their product got to them.

You'll see more refills, less extra cardboard, and more "here's exactly what we put in this" marketing as time goes on.

Social Media: Welcome to #PerfumeTok

Perfume used to be marketed with glossy ads featuring models on cliffs and horses on beaches. Now it's a person in their bedroom saying, "Okay, REAL TALK, this smells like your ex who finally went to therapy."

That shift changed everything.

Short videos made fragrance emotional and specific. "This smells like rich aunt energy." "Like a clean hoodie on someone you like." "Like walking into an expensive hotel lobby, you definitely can't afford."

Micro-influencers (small accounts, strong trust) move product. If you've watched someone talk about their acne or breakups for months, and then they say, "This is my comfort perfume," you listen.

Perfume became a hobby instead of a single "signature scent." People have "scent wardrobes," "perfume shelves," and "declutter" videos. They swap samples, rank the top 10 vanillas, and do blind-smell tests on their friends.

Gender rules loosened up. Men spray florals and talk about powdery scents. Women wear "men's" woods and leather. The bottle's label matters less than how it feels.

The good news: it's never been easier to find new perfumes. The not-so-good news: it's also easy to get caught up buying scents that work for someone else, not for you. Don't worry, we'll talk about how to keep both your wallet and your nose safe.

Arabian Fragrance Houses: Where Tradition Still Breathes

The Middle East has been the heartbeat of perfumery for what seems like forever. The world learned about oud, frankincense, myrrh, rose attars, and incense rituals. Today, several modern houses keep that heritage alive while speaking to a global audience.

Think of them as living proof that "luxury fragrance" isn't just a French thing.

1. Rasasi

A family-run house that grew from a single shop in Dubai into an international brand. Rasasi is known for:

Rich, long-lasting ouds and ambers.

Affordable blends that feel more expensive than they are.

A very "Arabian" approach to perfumery: bold, layered, meant to be felt.

They were early in the idea of mono-brand perfume stores—walk in, and you're in their world, not a mixed department store.

2. Swiss Arabian

Name says it all: Swiss precision + Arabian heritage.

Their scents mix Middle Eastern staples—oud, rose, saffron—with Western structures.

Result: approachable, but with a twist that feels different from mainstream mall fragrance.

3. Ajmal

Started with oud oil in India and built into a massive house across the Gulf.

Deep roots in agarwood (oud).

Wide catalog: traditional attars, modern blends, everything in between.

Still family-oriented, with a part of their profits going to community causes.

They show how a small, resource-based trade (wood resin) can turn into a whole story in bottles.

4. Amouage

The "haute couture" side of Arabian perfumery.

Founded in Oman at the royal request to preserve local fragrance art.

Known for rich, complex compositions—incense, frankincense, spices, florals.

Bottles and names nod to Omani culture and landscapes.

If you want to smell like a full novel, not just a short story, this is where people often look.

These houses are essential because they gently re-center the fragrance conversation. Instead of only looking to Paris for what's "refined," they remind everyone that the roots of perfumery run through the souks, mosques, markets, and homes of the Middle East.

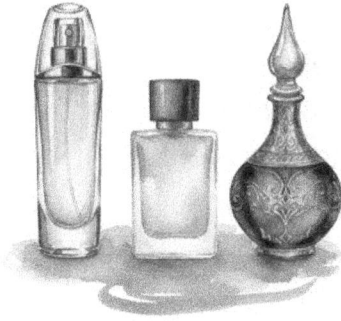

Dupe Houses: Luxury Vibes on a Regular Budget

On the other end of the spectrum, you have dupe brands—companies that create fragrances "inspired by" designer or niche perfumes but sell them at much lower prices.

The idea is simple: you don't have to spend rent money to smell like expensive vanilla, rose, or sandalwood.

Some key points about dupes:

They're entry points. If you're new to perfume, paying a smaller price to see if you even like a style can be a relief.

They change access. People who never set foot in a high-end boutique can now try versions of those scent profiles at home.

They spark debate. Critics say they sit too close to copying. Supporters argue that smell should not be reserved for the wealthy and that most perfumes are built on shared structures.

Many dupe brands:

Use straightforward packaging.

Focus on transparency and online reviews.

Offer both "inspired by" scents and original creations as they grow.

You'll also see brands like Zara making surprisingly good, affordable scents that echo famous perfumery trends. Are they identical? No. Are they often "close enough for real life?" For many people, yes.

Here's what matters: you get to enjoy whatever lets you join in. Wearing a $30 'inspired by' scent is just as real as wearing a $300 niche perfume. Both are just bottles of scented alcohol that make you feel something. The feeling is what counts, not the label.

Perfume as a Hobby: Shelves, Wardrobes, and Little Clouds of Joy

For some, perfume is like toothpaste. It's useful, necessary, and done. For others, it's a full-on hobby.

Signs you might be sliding into hobby territory:

You start saying "this one opens with..." like you're doing a wine tasting.

You know which friend loves clean musks, which loves gourmands, and which hates patchouli.

You can't remember the last time you finished a whole bottle, because you keep rotating.

Perfume collecting can look like:

Scent wardrobes. A few bottles for different moods: "interview," "beach," "date," "I need comfort," "I need to feel like a CEO."

Sample stashes. Little vials from indie brands, decants from friends, subscription boxes.

Community. Online groups where people swap samples, do blind swaps, and send each other "mystery vials" with handwritten clues.

It can also look like:

One or two special bottles are treated like treasure.

A wedding scent, an "I got the job" scent, a "this smells like my grandmother's house" scent.

All of this counts. At its best, perfume is low-stakes joy, a little luxury you tap onto your wrist on a rough Tuesday. It's a way to take up a bit of invisible space in a world that always wants you to shrink.

How to Choose Fragrances That Work for You

Okay, let's get practical. With all these options, how do you not drown?

Treat this as a loose guide, not a checklist you have to finish.

1. Start With Your Real Life

Before notes, before brands, look at:

Your climate. Hot? Humid? Dry? Freezing?

Your lifestyle. Office? Outdoors? Home with kids? Night shifts?

Your tolerance. Sensitive to strong smells? Migraines?

If you:

Work in healthcare or tight offices → you'll want lighter, closer-to-skin scents.

Live in heat and humidity → fresh, green, citrus, and light woods will probably feel better than dense ambers at noon.

Have fewer restrictions → you can play with strength and projection more.

2. Think About What You Already Love

Not perfume. Life.

What does your ideal morning smell like? Coffee, oranges, fresh laundry, rain?

What scents make you feel safe? Vanilla, baby powder, wood smoke, rose?

What scents make you feel energized? Mint, lemon, cut grass, salty air?

Jot down a quick list. That list will tell you more about what you like than any ad ever could.

3. Use Families as a Shortcut

Once you know "I love the smell of baking," that points you toward gourmands and vanilla.

If you love hiking and forests → woods, green, aromatic herbs.

If you love fresh laundry and hotels → musks, powdery notes, "clean" florals.

At a counter (or online):

Ask for samples in those families.

Don't try to smell 20 perfumes at once. Three to five at a time is more than enough.

Take paper strips but always test your favorites on skin.

4. Give Each Scent a Full Day

Perfume is a relationship, not a quick swipe left or right.

Spray your wrist.

Don't sniff for 10 minutes straight. Live. Do your day.

Check back:

Immediately (top notes)
30–60 minutes later (heart)
3–4 hours later (base)

Ask:

Do I like how it changes?
Did it give me a headache?
Did I forget about it entirely?
Did I keep catching whiffs and feeling happy?
If you're not sure right away, that's normal.
Some scents need a second try before you know
how you feel about them.

5.   Decide: Signature or Wardrobe?

There are two main styles:

Signature scent, people.

One main fragrance that becomes "your smell."
Clothes, scarves, and pillowcases all carry it.
People hug you and think, "Ah, that's them."

Wardrobe people.

A small collection: work scent, weekend scent, bedtime scent, date scent, comfort scent.

You don't have to pick one forever, but knowing where you lean helps you shop:

Signature route → invest in one bottle you genuinely love, maybe a travel size to keep in your bag, and ignore the noise.

Wardrobe route → build slowly, one type at a time (e.g., "Let me find my perfect fresh daytime scent first.").

6. Mix Price Points Without Shame

You are allowed to:

Wear an affordable dupe as your everyday scent and save the expensive bottle for events.

Pair a simple vanilla body mist with a pricier wood or floral.

Love a celebrity perfume more than anything niche.

Perfume isn't a test of your character.

7. Notice Your Gut

Sometimes, a scent makes you feel:
Taller.
Softer.
Calmer.
More "you."

Sometimes, it makes you feel awkward or "costumed," like you're wearing someone else's jacket.

Pay attention to that feeling. No review, no hype, no list of notes knows you better than your own gut.

The Future: Scent, Sustainability, and Self-Expression

Looking ahead, a few things are very likely:

More transparency. Brands will need to say more about ingredients, sourcing, and ethics. People care where their oils come from and who gets paid.

Refills and less waste. Refillable bottles, simpler boxes, less plastic. Old apothecary habits returning in modern packaging.

Less gender, more mood. "For him" and "for her" labels mean less. "For evening," "for comfort," "for focus," "for heat" might matter more.

More mixing. Layering lotions, oils, perfumes, and mists will stay popular because it lets people create something unique from everyday things.

More small stories. Niche houses, indie perfumers, and community brands will keep telling specific stories about one village, one childhood, one memory, and people will buy them because they want to feel something, not just smell "nice."

The heart of perfume is simple: people using scent to feel a little more alive.

Final Spritz: Smell as Story

Perfume lives in the invisible. You can't see it. You can't hold it. You only know it's there because it moves you or doesn't.

Think back through the journeys in this book:

Steam in a Moroccan hammam, carrying eucalyptus and black soap.

A grandmother in South Asia oiling her hair with jasmine or coconut.

Rice water dripping through long hair in a Chinese village.

Chebe powder combed into braids in the Sahel.

Vanilla-and-coffee scrubs in a Latin American kitchen.

A quick spritz before work in a small American bathroom.

Every one of those moments has a scent.

This chapter just gives you words for something your body already knows: smell is memory. Smell is mood. Smell is a kind of touch that doesn't need hands.

When you pick a fragrance, whether it's a fancy oud, a $30 vanilla dupe, a drugstore classic, or something from a tiny market stall, you're something great for yourself. You're choosing the mood you'll carry with you for the rest of your day.

You're saying:

"I want comfort."

"I want to feel sharp and awake."

"I want to feel mysterious."

"I want to feel like myself."

So spray on purpose. Or dab. Or roll a little oil on your wrists at night, even if you're the only one who'll notice. Take a slow breath and notice how you feel right then.

That's the actual ritual.

Not the brand name. Not the price. Not the review count.

Just you, your skin, your story, and a little cloud of scent that connects you to countless others doing the same thing under the same sky.

Wash. Glow. Spritz. Breathe. Repeat.

FINAL CHAPTER

Global Fusion – Rituals for a Connected World

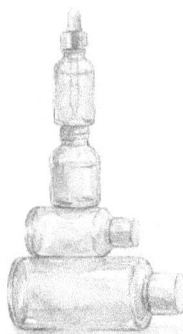

If you've made it this far, you've already gone further than most people ever do without even leaving your house. Basically, you've seen that every culture is saying the same thing in a different accent.

Take care of yourself.
Slow down for a moment.
Remember who you are.

That's the heart of beauty everywhere.

After digging into fragrance in Chapter 9, it's even more obvious. Scent tells a story. It brings back memories, changes your mood, and shapes how you see yourself way more than a mirror ever could. One smell can take you right back to a moment in your past. Another can help you determine who you want to be next. Perfume isn't just something you put on. It's a way in.

Now here's the thing.

These rituals might look different. From scrubbing with a Ghanaian net, soaking in a Finnish sauna, layering attars in the Middle East, or washing with rice water in Japan. However, they all come from the same place. People want to feel cared for so their minds can relax. That's something everyone understands. Think about a parent teaching a child to braid hair, a grandmother rubbing oil between her hands, or even someone online sharing a scent review just to make someone else happy. These moments matter.

This is just as true for the routines we have now. Even a regular shower can feel special if you pay attention. Washing your face at night can help you feel grounded when everything else feels out of control. Spraying on a scent you love can give you a lift, no explanation needed. These things aren't about vanity. They give your day some structure. They help you switch from morning to night, work to rest, or before to after. They remind you to slow down and feel human, even when life is moving fast.

Some routines stick with you for years. Some change as quickly as the latest trend. That's the good part about living in a linked world. You can try what works for you, let go of what doesn't, and create something that feels right for your life. Maybe your routine is a mix of your grandmother's advice, something you saw on TikTok, and a scent from a place you've never been but feel drawn to. That's not doing it wrong. That's just how things grow.

So here's the quiet truth I hope follows you after you close this book: Your routines are not chores. They're invitations.

Every time you wash your face, put on lotion, or spray a scent, you're giving yourself a little care. These small things help you feel grounded, even when you're tired. Your routines don't have to be fancy or take a lot of time. They just need to feel like yours. If you finish this book feeling more at home in your own skin, and a bit more connected to the world behind these traditions, then that's a win.

Let your routine be a soft place to land.
Let it shift with you.

Let it teach you who you are becoming.

And when you step out of the bathroom, scented or not, glowing or not, remember this one simple thing shared everywhere from Bali to Brooklyn:

The way you care for yourself becomes the way you carry yourself. That is your ritual now. And it's a beautiful one.

Sources & Inspiration

Everything in this book comes from a mix of places: history, culture, industry reports, and real-life traditions. Some of what I learned dives into the science and psychology of scent. Other parts come straight from beauty rituals that families and communities have passed down for generations. And a lot of it is about how fragrance and self-care keep changing right now. These sources shaped how I see things and what I wanted to share with you. I don't have all the answers, but I hope what you've read sparks your curiosity and helps you start your own journey.

References

Aftel, M. (2014). Fragrant: The secret life of scent. Riverhead Books.

Ayala, S. (2020). Perfume: The art and science of scent. HarperCollins.

Burr, C. (2008). The perfect scent: A year inside the perfume industry. Henry Holt.

Edwards, M. (2022). Fragrances of the world (34th ed.). Michael Edwards Publishing.

Hughes, G. (2019). Aromatic cultures: Global histories of fragrance. Routledge.

Le Guérer, A. (1992). Scent: The mysterious and essential powers of smell. Kodansha.

Miller, L. (2023). The psychology of fragrance use in the digital age. Journal of Consumer Culture, 18(4), 455–478.

Turner, L. (2018). Global bathing rituals: History, culture, and wellness. Oxford University Press.

Ullmann, L. (2021). The cultural evolution of perfume rituals. Anthropology Today, 37(2), 22–29.

World Perfumery Congress. (2023). A history of perfumery: From incense to innovation. WPC Press.

Further Reading

Ajmal Perfumes. (2025). About Ajmal. https://ensa.ajmal.com

Amouage. (2025). Company history and heritage. https://www.amouage.com

Blog Fragrance Oil. (2024). The rise of TikTok perfume culture. https://blog.fragrancesoil.com

Cosmopolitan. (2024). Fragrance wheel: Understanding scent families. https://www.cosmopolitan.com

Dossier. (2025). Brand mission and product development. https://www.dossier.co

Dyer, M. (2020). Cultural beauty rituals around the world. Harper & Row.

Edwards, M. (2019). Fragrances of the world. Fragrances of the World Press.

Fashion Magazine. (2024). Global fragrance market: Trending notes and consumer behavior. https://www.fashionmagazine.com

Fresh Beauty Fix. (2023). How to choose and layer fragrances. https://freshbeautyfix.com

Glimpse, The Research Platform. (2025). Fragrance trend report: Sustainability, dupes, & Gen Z shifts. https://meetglimpse.com

Jafza. (2024). Rasasi Perfumes: Brand overview. https://jafza.ae

Ramsons Perfumes. (2025). Fragrance trends: Notes and directions. https://ramsonsperfumes.com

Rasasi. (2024). Company history and production overview. https://www.rasasi.com

Swiss Arabian. (2024). Brand history. https://uae.swissarabian.com

Tache, S. (2024). Democratizing luxury: The rise of accessible fragrance. Medium. https://medium.com

TikTok Fragrance Analytics. (2024). Viral scent trends and digital influence. https://www.tiktok.com

Vogue. (2024). How scent layering became a global beauty ritual. https://www.vogue.com

Zara Fragrances. (2023). Modern interpretations of classic scents. https://www.zara.com

About Nadia

Nadia Kessyn writes about beauty, self-care, and fragrance, but not in the way you might think. She pays attention to small routines like washing your face, choosing a scent, caring for your body, and asks a simple question: Why hurry through these moments when they could mean something more? Nadia brings together stories and research to show how these everyday habits are shaped by culture and tradition. She makes rituals from around the world feel close and familiar, not out of reach.

When Nadia isn't writing, she's reading, noticing the small things, or wondering how people care for themselves in different corners of the world. She knows self-care doesn't have to be fancy. It doesn't have to be complicated. What matters is the intention, not perfection. Her hope is simple: to help you find small rituals that feel good and help you feel more connected to the world around you.

www.ingramcontent.com/pod-product-compliance
Lightning Source LLC
Chambersburg PA
CBHW031207270326
41931CB00006B/445